High Blood Pressure

FOR

DUMMIES®

2ND EDITION

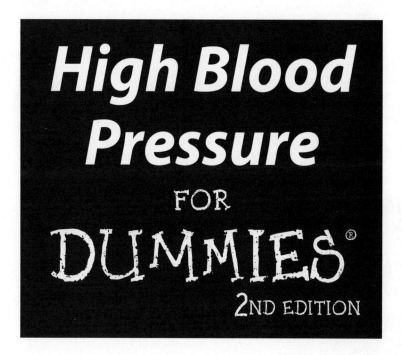

High Blood Pressure

FOR

DUMMIES®

2ND EDITION

by Alan L. Rubin, MD

BICENTENNIAL
1807
WILEY
2007
BICENTENNIAL

Wiley Publishing, Inc.

High Blood Pressure For Dummies,® 2nd Edition

Published by
Wiley Publishing, Inc.
111 River St.
Hoboken, NJ 07030-5774
www.wiley.com

WILEY

About the Author

Alan L. Rubin, MD has been managing and studying high blood pressure for three decades. He is a bestselling author whose previous books, *Diabetes For Dummies, Diabetes Cookbook For Dummies,* and *Thyroid For Dummies,* have been major successes. Letters of praise from numerous readers verify the important role that his books have played in their lives. The books have been translated into seven languages, and there are special editions for the United Kingdom, Canada, and Australia. His books provide the latest information on every aspect of their subject while being written in an easy-to-understand format that's full of humor and wisdom.

Dr. Rubin has practiced endocrinology in San Francisco since 1973. He teaches doctors, medical students, and nonprofessionals through classes, lectures, and articles. He has been on numerous radio and television shows, answering questions about diabetes, thyroid disease, and high blood pressure. He serves as a consultant to many pharmaceutical companies and companies that make products for high blood pressure.

Dr. Rubin discusses many health issues in the numerous "Healthcasts" that he has recorded, which may be heard or downloaded at his Web site, www.drrubin.com.

Dedication

This book is dedicated to my mother, Edith. Besides the fact that I would not exist were it not for her (with a little help from my father, Julius), she always let me know in no uncertain terms that I could do anything I set my mind to. This is the fourth *For Dummies* book I have written, and that knowledge helped to get me through each one. Not only did she give me total verbal approval, but she backed it up by making sure I got a great undergraduate education at Brandeis University and medical education at New York University School of Medicine. Most important of all, she made sure I knew that I was loved.

Author's Acknowledgments

Unlike a baby, this book has more than two parents. The people who worked on it are dedicated, bright, and cheerful, and they deserve a standing ovation. The original concept belongs to Kathy Nebenhaus, who was Lifestyles Publisher when the first edition began and is now Vice President of Professional and Trade Publishing at Wiley Books. Acquisitions Editor Michael Lewis was tremendously helpful throughout the writing of the book, smoothing all the rough edges that inevitably surround such a major project. Project Editor Georgette Beatty had a very clear idea of how the book would best serve its readers and offered many helpful suggestions to accomplish this. Copy Editor Pam Ruble made sure that my words, my sentences, and my paragraphs followed the rules of the English language. Last but definitely not least, Myron H. Weinberger, MD, was the technical editor for this book, utilizing his great knowledge of this subject to assure that my information is consistent with current medical practice. To all of them, I owe major thanks.

Publisher's Acknowledgments

We're proud of this book; please send us your comments through our Dummies online registration form located at www.dummies.com/register/.

Some of the people who helped bring this book to market include the following:

Acquisitions, Editorial, and Media Development

Project Editor: Georgette Beatty

(Previous Edition: Alissa Schwipps)

Acquisitions Editor: Michael Lewis

Copy Editor: Pam Ruble

(Previous Edition: Esmeralda St. Clair)

Technical Editor: Myron H. Weinberger, MD

Editorial Manager: Michelle Hacker

Editorial Assistants: Erin Calligan Mooney, Joe Niesen, Leeann Harney

Cover Photo: © Dynamic Graphics

Cartoons: Rich Tennant (www.the5thwave.com)

Composition Services

Project Coordinator: Jennifer Theriot

Layout and Graphics: Carl Byers, Joyce Haughey, Stephanie D. Jumper, Heather Ryan, Erin Zeltner

Special Art: Illustrations by Kathryn Born, MA

Anniversary Logo Design: Richard Pacifico

Proofreaders: Laura Albert, John Greenough, Aptara

Indexer: Potomac Indexing, LLC

Publishing and Editorial for Consumer Dummies

Diane Graves Steele, Vice President and Publisher, Consumer Dummies

Joyce Pepple, Acquisitions Director, Consumer Dummies

Kristin A. Cocks, Product Development Director, Consumer Dummies

Michael Spring, Vice President and Publisher, Travel

Kelly Regan, Editorial Director, Travel

Publishing for Technology Dummies

Andy Cummings, Vice President and Publisher, Dummies Technology/General User

Composition Services

Gerry Fahey, Vice President of Production Services

Debbie Stailey, Director of Composition Services

Contents at a Glance

Table of Contents

Introduction

*W*hen I was growing up, my mother often used the pressure cooker to make dinner in a hurry. The idea was that under higher pressure, the food got done faster. High blood pressure in people is like that. If you permit yourself to have high blood pressure, you'll get done faster too. What do I mean by *done?* I'm talking about all the medical complications like heart attack, stroke, and kidney failure — and the shortened life span.

High blood pressure, or *hypertension,* as doctors like to call it, affects more than 65 million adults in the United States and between 15 and 25 percent of the rest of the world, according to the World Health Organization. This means that when you're in a room with four other adults, one of the four of you probably has high blood pressure. One major problem is that a third of the people who have high blood pressure don't know it; the disease is generally free of symptoms until it's had time to do damage (over ten or more years). And that's why high blood pressure is often known as the *silent killer.*

One source of optimism is that more than half of the other two-thirds who know they have high blood pressure are now receiving adequate treatment (37 percent of all people with blood pressure, up from the 27 percent I noted in my first edition). This means 16 percent of those who know they have high blood pressure are still inadequately treated and another 15 percent of them are untreated. Specialists don't know exactly why there are still so many untreated and inadequately treated, but we know this book wasn't around when the last set of statistics was gathered.

Translating percentages into numbers, around 41 million Americans are at risk from the complications of high blood pressure because of inadequate treatment, no treatment, or lack of awareness that they have the disease. The situation in most other countries is even worse.

For decades, the crusade to bring this vast problem under control seemed to be making great progress because the occurrence of strokes seemed to be declining. Although that control deteriorated for a while as the frequency of strokes increased, now we're headed in the right direction again. The trouble is that the overall number of adults and children with high blood pressure is increasing as the population ages and gets heavier. Major investments of time, energy, and money are needed to deal with the millions of people still not receiving adequate blood pressure control.

Like diabetes, high blood pressure is a lifestyle disease. It tends to occur in more affluent nations, where food is plentiful and hard manual labor is less common. This fact is both a problem and a challenge. On the one hand, affluent societies don't want to give up their benefits. On the other, these more fortunate folks don't want to destroy themselves.

In this book, you can find everything you need to know about high blood pressure — its causes, its consequences, and its treatment. You'll soon realize that high blood pressure is easy to recognize and just as easy to treat. Sure, great drugs are available for treating high blood pressure, but drugs inevitably come with side effects, a price tag, and doctor visits. Far safer and less costly is a dedication on your part to prevention — changing the lifestyle habits that lead to high blood pressure. You can find all the necessary information on how to make these changes as you read the chapters of this book, especially Part III.

I always like to have a bottom line in my books, and this one is no exception. The bottom line is this: You never have to suffer any of the consequences of high blood pressure. You have it within your brain and within your body to prevent or successfully treat high blood pressure. Imagine if all the people with high blood pressure heeded this advice and got theirs under control. Each year about 275,000 lives would be saved and a much larger number would be spared a life of suffering from its consequences. And that's just in the United States, not to mention the rest of the world!

If you've read any of my previous books, *Diabetes For Dummies, Diabetes Cookbook For Dummies,* or *Thyroid For Dummies,* you know that I use humor to get my point across, a technique that characterizes the *For Dummies* series. I want to emphasize that I'm not trying to trivialize anyone's suffering by being comic about it. In fact, Norman Cousins, who wrote *Anatomy of an Illness as Perceived by the Patient* (Bantam Doubleday Dell), showed how he cured himself of an *incurable* disease using humor, and other writers have shown that humor has healing properties. A positive attitude — far more than a negative one — is conducive to a positive outcome.

About This Book

Since the last edition of this book, big changes have occurred in our understanding of high blood pressure and its treatment. The categories of high blood pressure have been reduced, and our recommendations about early treatment have changed as well. New drugs are available and old ones are off the market. A major Medicare drug plan, Part D, has confused millions of elderly Americans and changed how they pay for their drugs, including those for high blood pressure. These changes alone are more than enough justification for a new edition of *High Blood Pressure For Dummies.*

This edition has more emphasis on prevention. I also include new discoveries and myths about high blood pressure, so if you already have the first edition, know that I've packed this one with new stuff. (At the very least, buy it for your spouse — then borrow it so you stay up to date!)

But the main reason I wanted to write this update comes from an article that appears in the January 2007 issue of the journal *Diabetes Care.* The article points out that "despite the publication of increasingly aggressive guidelines for lowering blood pressure, [high blood pressure] remains substantially unimproved among diabetic patients." In other words, the number of people with diabetes is increasing explosively, but they're not achieving the level of blood pressure control that will prevent heart attacks, strokes, and amputations. I hope to change this outcome by helping the even larger population without diabetes to control their blood pressure.

Even with all the new information in this edition, no one expects you to read it cover to cover. Because the first few chapters are a general introduction to high blood pressure, you may want to start in Part I, but if you prefer to go right to the treatment or the special concerns of different populations, by all means, do so.

You'll notice that each chapter stands alone — you don't have to skip back to Chapter 3 to understand Chapter 12, and you don't have to start at the beginning to understand the end. This book's not a novel (though high blood pressure does make a pretty convincing villain!); it's a tool to help you manage your high blood pressure.

Conventions Used in This Book

I'd love to use all nonscientific terms in this book, but if I did, you and your doctor would be speaking two different languages. So I use the scientific terms, but I explain them with simple language the first time you see them.

As for the synonymous terms *high blood pressure* and *hypertension,* I use the simpler term — high blood pressure — in all cases. This choice seems to be the trend, and I think it's a good one.

Here are a few additional conventions that I use to guide you through this book:

- *Italics* point out defined terms and emphasize certain words.
- **Boldface** text highlights key words in bulleted lists and actions to take in numbered steps.
- Monofont indicates Web addresses.

When this book was printed, some Web addresses may have needed to break across two lines of text. If that happened, rest assured that I haven't put in any extra characters (such as hyphens) to indicate the break. So, when using one of these Web addresses, just type exactly what you see in this book, pretending that the line break doesn't exist.

What You're Not to Read

Throughout the book, shaded areas *(sidebars)* contain material that's interesting but not essential to your understanding. If you don't care to go so deeply into a subject, skip the sidebars. You'll still understand everything else.

Foolish Assumptions

This book makes no assumptions about what you know. Key points are always marked clearly, and I explain all new terms. But if you already know a great deal, you'll still find new information that adds to your knowledge. You probably fall into one of the following categories:

- You've been diagnosed with high blood pressure but haven't started treatment.
- You're being treated for high blood pressure but aren't happy with the results.
- You have a close friend or family member with high blood pressure.

How This Book Is Organized

The book is divided into six parts to help you find out all you want to know about high blood pressure.

Part I: Understanding High Blood Pressure

This part is really the introduction to the subject of high blood pressure. You discover the definition of high blood pressure, how to measure it correctly, and how to separate *essential* (that is, from unknown causes) high blood pressure from *secondary* high blood pressure (from another disease). You also discover the risk factors that increase your chances of developing high blood pressure.

Part II: Considering the Medical Consequences

High blood pressure can damage many parts of the body, but it's especially dangerous to your heart, kidneys, and brain. In this part, you find out exactly how the damage occurs and how it affects these important organs.

Part III: Treating (Or Preventing) High Blood Pressure

In this part, I introduce everything we know about preventing high blood pressure and lowering high blood pressure after it develops. This condition is highly treatable, but first you need to know you have it and then you need to know what to do about it. High blood pressure treatment has definite goals that you must meet; you can't just take a pill and assume you're home free.

Part IV: Taking Care of Special Populations

Three groups of people (pregnant women, children, and the elderly) deserve special consideration because high blood pressure acts differently and has different consequences for them. This part addresses their problems.

Part V: The Part of Tens

Like many other major medical conditions, misinformation about high blood pressure is rampant. In the Part of Tens, I clear up some of it (not all, because it accumulates faster than I can address it!) and show you how to take simple measures to control your blood pressure.

Just to whet your appetite and convince you that the field's advancing by leaps and bounds, I also provide ten new up-to-the-minute discoveries.

Appendix

New discoveries are going to make even this new edition obsolete after several years. For this reason, I want you to know the best resources for the latest information. More and more, this means the Internet. If you're still not connected to the World Wide Web, get with it! It's like having the world's libraries at your fingertips.

Icons Used in This Book

Books in the *For Dummies* series feature icons that direct you toward information of particular interest or importance. Here's an explanation of this book's icons:

This icon signals information important enough to get the advice or assistance of your doctor.

This icon means the information is essential. Be sure you understand it.

This icon points out important information that can save you time and energy.

Take this icon seriously. It warns against potential problems (for example, mixing the wrong drugs).

Where to Go from Here

Where you go from here depends on your needs. Want to understand how high blood pressure develops? Head to Part I. If you or someone you know has a complication due to high blood pressure, skip to Part II. For help in treating high blood pressure (or preventing it entirely), turn to Part III. If you're pregnant or have a child or parent with high blood pressure, Part IV is your next stop. For a bird's-eye view of treatment, high blood pressure mythology, and the latest discoveries, check out Part V.

If you've experienced something funny in connection with your high blood pressure, my e-mail is highbloodpressure@drrubin.com. By all means, let me know the situation. And if it's appropriate, I'll share it with the world in a future edition of this book.

In any case, as my mother used to say when she gave me a present, use this book in good health.

Part I

Understanding High Blood Pressure

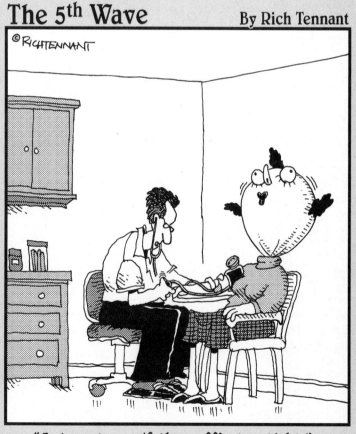

"Let me know if the cuff's too tight."

In this part . . .

What are those two numbers your doctor gives you after measuring your blood pressure? In this part, I answer that question and describe the correct technique for taking blood pressure at home or in your doctor's office. I also discuss who is most at risk for developing high blood pressure and what you need to know about secondary high blood pressure.

Chapter 1

Introducing High Blood Pressure

*I*f you have high blood pressure, you're in good (though not terribly healthy) company. Sixty-five million Americans (one in three adults) have high blood pressure. A list of the people in this country with high blood pressure would read like a *Who's Who*. The problem is that, without proper treatment, many of those people will be on a list of *Who Was Who* sooner than they expect. The reason is that high blood pressure is the largest risk factor for heart attacks, brain attacks (strokes), and disease of the arteries. Don't let yourself or a loved one get on that second list without a fight!

You can do so much about high blood pressure — you can prevent it, and if it's already high, you can control it. But before you act, you need to know what high blood pressure is and how you measure it. You also need up-to-date information about its causes and its treatments. This book is your blood pressure companion, providing you with a solid understanding of your blood pressure: how it affects your body organ by organ, who is at risk, how you can prevent it, and how you can treat it after it's properly diagnosed.

As you'll discover, a few simple alterations to your lifestyle can prevent high blood pressure. My hope is that as you read this book, you're spurred on to make these changes, not just now but in the future. High blood pressure is a chronic disease. You may lower your blood pressure in the short term, but the goal is long-term control to prevent other medical consequences (see Part II).

Take charge of your blood pressure now so you don't suffer the fate of a health-food storeowner who posted a sign saying, "Closed due to illness."

Understanding Your Cardiovascular System

To understand how elevated blood pressure affects your overall health, you need to understand the contribution of your heart and blood vessels. Your cardiovascular system — your heart, arteries, veins, capillaries, and the blood that fills them — nourishes your body and connects each part to every other part. The cardiovascular system carries

- **Food** (carbohydrates, protein, fat, vitamins, and minerals) from the gastrointestinal tract to every organ in the body
- **Oxygen** from the lungs and in the blood to distant organs
- **Waste,** a normal product of your body's metabolism

  For example, the cardiovascular system carries carbon dioxide to the lungs and the other waste products to the liver and kidneys.

Pressure must exist to push the blood through the cardiovascular system. (Otherwise your blood would pool in your legs due to gravity when you stood up!) Just as your household water supply reaches a faucet because of pressure pushing it through the pipes, blood reaches your brain because pressure is allowing it to defy gravity and rise from the heart.

The heart muscle (the source of this pressure) squeezes out the blood forcefully so the blood not only defies gravity but also travels through the smallest passageways (the capillaries).

When essential body organs like the kidneys don't receive enough pressure to function properly, they signal the heart to pump harder. But what's good for the kidneys may not be good for the brain or the blood vessels themselves. And that's when the consequences of high blood pressure occur (see Part II).

Measuring Your Pressure and Understanding the Measurement

When the nurse in your doctor's office measures your blood pressure, she puts the contraption with a cuff, a gauge, and some Velcro around your arm. She pumps the cuff up with air, listens with the stethoscope, turns a screw to release the air pressure, and then writes down a couple of numbers in your chart. Then your doctor enters and says those numbers are "good" or "not so good."

What's that contraption? What's the meaning of those numbers? Why do they seem to have such a profound effect on your life? Good questions. The contraption is a *sphygmomanometer.* When your doctor reads the numbers, say *135 over 85,* the first number is the *systolic blood pressure,* and the second number is the *diastolic blood pressure.* In Chapter 2, I discuss what these two pressures measure, what their numbers mean, and why the results have such a serious effect on your life.

One of the most effective steps you can take in understanding your health is to measure your own blood pressure with a home monitoring device. I cover this topic extensively in Chapter 2 as well.

Looking at the Risk Factors for High Blood Pressure

Researchers have made tremendous efforts to understand the cause of high blood pressure and which populations are at risk of developing the disease. They know that numerous unalterable factors affect blood pressure (age, sex, ethnic background, and family history) and, to some extent, *how* these factors contribute to high blood pressure. But they still don't know which of these factors is the most important. I discuss risk factors in detail in Chapter 3.

Certain changeable factors (such as diet, exercise routine, and stress) can also place you at risk of developing high blood pressure. Ask yourself the following questions:

- ✔ Am I less active than I could be in my day-to-day routine?
- ✔ Am I overweight?
- ✔ Do I eat many salty foods?
- ✔ Do I have a stressful lifestyle?
- ✔ Do I smoke? Drink?

If you answer "Yes" to any one of these questions, then you're at risk of developing high blood pressure. The more questions that you answer in the affirmative, the greater your odds are for developing high blood pressure. But if you decrease the stress in your life and keep a rein on these changeable factors, you can decrease the possibility of developing high blood pressure. I discuss high blood pressure prevention further in Chapter 3.

Research indicates that high blood pressure arises in two stages:

- ✔ **A primary cause** such as the increased blood volume or constriction of the blood vessels: At this stage, high blood pressure is reversible.

> ✔ **A secondary result** such as the blood vessels permanently thickening: At this stage, high blood pressure becomes irreversible without the use of potent drugs.

Ninety-five percent of high blood pressure is categorized *essential high blood pressure* (but *primary high blood pressure* would be a better term); the cause is unknown. The remaining cases are *secondary high blood pressure;* a specific disease is identified as the cause. When that disease is treated, the blood pressure usually returns to normal. I discuss some causes of secondary high blood pressure in Chapter 4.

Focusing on the Consequences of High Blood Pressure

If untreated, your high blood pressure can wreak havoc on your heart, kidneys, and brain.

> ✔ Heart attacks or heart failure may be the major consequence for your heart (see Chapter 5).
>
> ✔ Kidney failure may eliminate the filtering function of your kidneys (see Chapter 6).
>
> ✔ A brain attack (stroke) may destroy important brain tissue and the movements it controls in the body (see Chapter 7).

Deaths due to these conditions do occur, but the great majority of people who have serious conditions from high blood pressure suffer debilitating illness. Of those who survive a massive heart attack, kidney failure, or brain attack, many require the care of other people for the rest of their lives.

Most of this sickness and death due to high blood pressure is preventable, and Part III gives you all the tools you need to minimize those risks. The process may cost you time and resources, but the freedom from illness and the prospect of a longer life are well worth the effort.

Lowering High Blood Pressure with Different Treatments

Treating high blood pressure (or preventing it entirely) involves all the tools I discuss in Part III. Get started with the following guidelines and check out Chapter 8 for an outline of a successful plan:

Connecting cardiac output and peripheral resistance

An increase in blood *volume* (the amount of blood in the blood vessels) creates an increase in *cardiac output* (the amount of blood that the heart squeezes out with each heartbeat). For example, an increase in blood volume may result from salt intake, which then causes water retention. Because the body doesn't permit the cardiac output to remain elevated, it lowers the output by increasing the *peripheral resistance* (the blood vessels constrict, reducing the amount of blood flowing through the tissues). This rise in peripheral resistance leads to increased blood pressure.

A minor alteration in body chemistry may be enough to cause persistent high blood pressure. For example, a slight increase in *angiotensin II* (a hormone produced when the kidney detects a low blood pressure) may cause thickening and narrowing of the blood vessels that leads to sustained high blood pressure. Other hormones, called *growth factors,* can lead to narrow arteries and increased peripheral resistance as well.

On the other hand, *nitric oxide* (a chemical made in the endothelial cells that line the inside of the blood vessels) is the most potent cause of *widening* blood vessels. If anything blocks the production of nitric oxide, the blood pressure rises. And because nitric oxide is reduced in *essential* (unknown causes) high blood pressure, this reduction may be an additional cause of increased peripheral resistance.

1. **Switch from a diet that promotes high blood pressure to a diet that lowers blood pressure** (see Chapters 9 and 10).

2. **Eliminate the poisons like tobacco, excessive alcohol, and some caffeine** (see Chapter 11).

3. **Add regular exercise** (see Chapter 12).

Just these three steps may be enough to lower your pressure to normal. If not, you have the option of adding one or more drugs (see Chapter 13). *Note:* Drugs aren't *substitutes;* they're *additions* to lifestyle changes.

Protecting Children, Pregnant Women, and the Elderly

Special factors must be considered when evaluating and treating high blood pressure in children, pregnant women, and the elderly:

✔ The elderly (see Chapter 14) usually have other complicating diseases, are taking many other medications, and may have special dietary requirements.

✔ Children (see Chapter 15) are growing, maturing, and subject to the problems of relating to their peers; kids certainly don't want to be sick or even labeled as *sick*. Diagnosis and treatment of high blood pressure in children is challenging to say the least.

✔ Throughout pregnancy, a woman is making new hormones while her body undergoes major changes. The high blood pressure that occasionally develops as a direct complication of pregnancy can harm both a mother and her unborn baby (see Chapter 16).

Staying Informed

The Part of Tens chapters in this book give you helpful tips on reducing your blood pressure and debunking blood pressure myths.

✔ In Chapter 17, you can find ten simple ways to prevent or reduce blood pressure. Individually, they each help to lower the pressure by a few millimeters of mercury. But taken together, they help you avoid the medical complications of high blood pressure. You can add them to your lifestyle one at a time or several at once — if you're up to it.

✔ In Chapter 18 I take on ten or so myths about high blood pressure and its treatment that are the most popular *and* the most detrimental to your health. (If you know of a myth that you think is damaging to many people with high blood pressure, by all means e-mail me at highbloodpressure@drrubin.com and let me know.)

✔ As in all fields of medicine that affect large numbers of people, the research on high blood pressure is enormous and ongoing. Chapter 19 introduces some of the latest information that may save your life.

Finally, the book has a publication deadline date. Discoveries made after that date can't be in this edition (but will be in a future one). To keep up with future developments, the appendix provides the best places to look for new information. Some of that info is also on my Web site (www.drrubin.com) or linked to it (click on the Web addresses in the *high blood pressure* section).

All this material comes to you at a bargain price. As the sign on the farmer's gate reads: "The farmer allows walkers to cross the field for free but the bull charges."

Chapter 2

Detecting High Blood Pressure

• •

• •

Measuring blood pressure correctly is key to diagnosing high blood pressure. You or another trained individual can take that measurement. This chapter shows you how to take that measurement because everything that follows will depend on its accuracy. If you notice that your healthcare provider isn't measuring your blood pressure accurately, don't hesitate to tell him. It's your life, your health, and your future that I'm talking about.

Much goes into an accurate blood pressure measurement. It requires a properly working instrument, a patient who is physically and mentally prepared for the measurement, and someone who knows how to measure blood pressure properly. And after it's done properly, it needs to be repeated to be sure of the numbers.

Following a diagnosis of high blood pressure, the evaluation process determines whether there is a *secondary* cause for the high blood pressure (that is, a definite disease that brings it on; see Chapter 4). I provide that proper evaluation at the end of this chapter so you can confirm that no stone is left unturned.

Focusing on Blood Pressure Gauge Fundamentals

The instrument that measures your blood pressure is a *sphygmomanometer* (pronounced sfig-mo-ma-*nom*-et-er — so why don't they spell it that way?). However, I think *blood pressure gauge* is clearer and easier to pronounce. I hope you don't mind if I call it that from now on.

The blood pressure gauge consists of a cuff that goes around your arm above the elbow. The *bladder* is the part of the cuff that fills with air. A tube connects the cuff to a column of mercury (that looks like an outdoor thermometer) at one end and a rubber bulb at the other. When the rubber bulb is squeezed, the air pressure in this closed system forces the column of mercury to rise as the bladder fills with air. Numbers along the column of mercury indicate how much pressure is present.

The mercury blood pressure gauge is the gold standard for blood pressure measurement. Very little can cause this device to malfunction because the column of mercury is the only moving part. *Note:* The mercury blood pressure gauge is becoming less common because mercury is toxic and has the potential to contaminate the environment.

An alternative blood pressure gauge that's rising in popularity is the *aneroid* blood pressure gauge — a spring-gauge model that uses air pressure to move a needle on a scale. Each degree the needle moves represents one millimeter of mercury. This gauge is inexpensive and easier to transport than the mercury blood pressure gauge. Figure 2-1 shows both mercury and aneroid blood pressure gauges.

Mercury blood pressure gauge

Aneroid blood pressure gauge

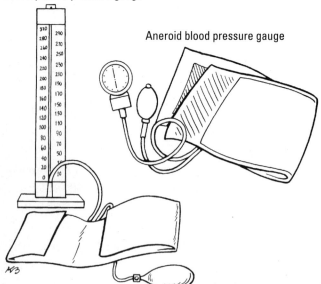

Figure 2-1:
Mercury
and aneroid
blood
pressure
gauges.

Both models require a certain degree of upkeep.

✔ Mercury blood pressure gauge: Check periodically to be sure the top of the column is at zero before pressure is added and that the mercury moves freely.

✔ Aneroid blood pressure gauge: Calibrate and validate it on a regular basis at your doctor's office (at least every six months) by attaching it to the pressure system of a mercury manometer. The gauges should read the same pressure when air is introduced.

Unlike the mercury gauge, the aneroid gauge has many parts that can wear down after a period of time. But according to a Mayo Clinic study in the March 2001 *Archives of Internal Medicine,* "Well-maintained aneroid devices are an accurate and useful alternative [to mercury devices]."

Taking Your Blood Pressure Correctly

Your blood pressure can be taken with a mercury blood pressure gauge, an aneroid manometer, or an electronic device for measuring the blood pressure, so long as the device has been recently calibrated and validated. (For more on the differences between mercury and aneroid blood pressure gauges, see the previous section. I discuss electronic gauges in the "Taking Your Blood Pressure at Home" section later in this chapter.)

Don't use blood pressure gauges in supermarkets or pharmacies; they're rarely well maintained.

Follow these few simple rules to get an accurate reading:

✔ **Don't smoke or drink alcohol or coffee within 15 minutes of a blood pressure measurement.**

✔ **The length of the bladder should be 80 percent of the circumference of the upper arm.** This means that heavy or very muscular people with thick arms need a larger bladder, while children need a smaller bladder.

✔ **Your posture and actions are important:**

- Sit with your back and arm supported; your supported elbow should be at about the level of your heart.

- Keep your legs from dangling.

- Rest for several minutes in that position before the measurement.

- Remain silent during the measurement.

To take the reading, follow these numbered steps:

1. **Place the cuff over your bare arm, leaving the cuff's lower edge about an inch above the bend of the elbow. Close the cuff around the arm, and then stick the Velcro together at the ends of the cuff.**

2. **Place the earpieces of the stethoscope in your ears and place the stethoscope *bell* at the side of the cuff away from your heart and over the *brachial* artery (in the inner area of your bent elbow; see Figure 2-2).**

   The stethoscope is a convenient device to listen for sounds at various body sites; its *bell* is the point of contact. The two earpieces at the other end of the stethoscope enable the individual taking the measurement to hear the steady thump in the brachial artery.

3. **Tighten the screw at the side of the gauge's rubber bulb and then squeeze the bulb.** Air is pumped into the bulb, and the cuff expands until the blood flow through your brachial artery stops.

   The pressure in the cuff rapidly increases to 30 millimeters of mercury above that point. No sound can be heard in the stethoscope and no pulse can be felt in the wrist.

4. **Turn the screw again, this time loosening the valve in the bulb and lessening the air pressure.** Pressure decreases at the rate of 2 millimeters per second. Blood begins to flow through the artery again.

5. **When you hear the first sound in the stethoscope, note the number beside the top of the mercury column.** This first sound in the stethoscope is the *systolic blood pressure* (SBP), the first number in the blood pressure reading. (See the "Understanding the Numbers" section later in this chapter.)

6. **When the sound ceases, note the number beside the top of the mercury column.** At this point, the cuff decompresses and blood flows freely in the artery. This is the *diastolic blood pressure* (DBP), the second number in the blood pressure reading. (See the "Understanding the Numbers" section later in this chapter.)

7. **Record the SBP and the DBP numbers immediately (don't depend on memory) and note which arm (right or left) you used.**

8. **If the first measurement is above 140 systolic or 90 diastolic, take another measurement in the same arm after 60 seconds. Then measure the other arm.**

   In the future, use the arm that has the higher blood pressure (although they're often the same). The *average* of the two measurements in the arm that supplies the higher readings is the correct blood pressure.

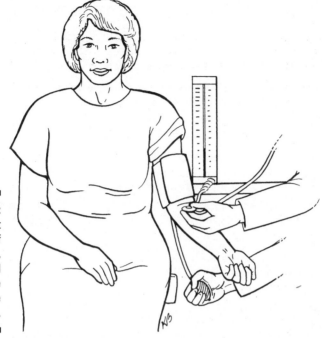

Figure 2-2:
The correct position of the patient, the blood pressure cuff, and the stethoscope.

Also measure the blood pressure while the patient is in a standing position, especially if the patient experiences lightheadedness on standing. If a fall of 20 or more millimeters of mercury occurs in systolic blood pressure or 10 or more in diastolic blood pressure, the patient has *orthostatic hypotension,* an abnormally great fall in blood pressure with standing.

If your blood pressure isn't normal, don't start any treatment on the basis of one office visit. This is treatment for life and should begin only after confirmation at a second and even a third office visit. As I show in the next section, your blood pressure in your doctor's office may not be an accurate assessment of your blood pressure despite entirely correct techniques. ***Note:*** A blood pressure reading greater than 180/120 millimeters of mercury (mm *Hg,* the chemical notation for mercury) requires immediate treatment.

Avoiding an Inaccurate Reading

Because your reading can mean the difference between a lifetime of taking pills and freedom from such a task, you want to avoid the many problems that may lead to an inaccurate blood pressure reading. Such problems can arise at every stage of taking a measurement as a result of equipment failures, faulty observation, or patient difficulties. Remember the points in the next two sections whenever your blood pressure is measured.

Steering clear of equipment problems

A faulty stethoscope can lead to an inaccurate blood pressure reading. To get a good reading, make sure

- The earpieces aren't plugged and sound can be heard clearly. If the earpieces are broken, replace them.

- The bell of the stethoscope (the part that's placed on the arm) is not cracked.

- The stethoscope includes an acceptable length of tubing (usually 22 to 28 inches) between the bell and the earpieces. Tubing that's too long may diminish the sound so it can't be heard.

To ensure an accurate reading when using a mercury blood pressure gauge, make sure

- The top of the column of mercury registers at zero when the blood pressure gauge has no air pressure.

- The column of mercury is vertical.

- The tubing is clean and unobstructed. If you disconnect the tubing, you should be able to blow air through it. If the air doesn't flow freely, get new tubing.

- The size of the cuff *(bladder)* is correct.

    - A cuff that's too narrow for the patient's arm gives a high reading.

    - A cuff that's too wide for the patient's arm gives a low reading.

Sidestepping faulty observation and patient problems

To avoid faulty observation, make sure

- The person taking your blood pressure doesn't allow a preconceived notion of your blood pressure to influence the reading.

- The person who measures your blood pressure writes down your reading rather than memorizing it. Poor memory often leads to an inaccurate charting of the numbers.

To avoid patient problems and ensure an accurate blood pressure reading, make sure

- ✔ The blood pressure cuff is at heart level. If the cuff is above heart level, the reading may be inaccurately low. If the cuff is below heart level, the reading may be inaccurately high.

- ✔ The patient's back is supported and his legs aren't dangling. He should be in a chair, not on an exam table.

- ✔ If the patient has a large, muscular arm (that may cause an inaccurately high reading), you use a blood pressure gauge with a cuff that's large enough to accommodate the arm.

- ✔ If the patient has calcified arteries (common among the elderly) that are hard to compress, you use another method of blood pressure measurement like direct insertion of a blood pressure gauge into the artery.

Whew! You have quite a few factors to keep in mind while taking your blood pressure. After you have an accurate reading, it's time to process the information. Read on for more about the meaning of those numbers.

Understanding the Numbers

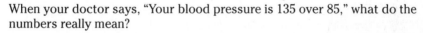

When your doctor says, "Your blood pressure is 135 over 85," what do the numbers really mean?

- ✔ The first number is the *systolic blood pressure* (SBP), the amount of pressure in your arteries as the heart pumps. *Systole* is the rhythmic contraction of your heart muscle when it's expelling blood from your left ventricle — the large chamber on the left side of your heart. The *aortic valve* sits between that chamber and your *aorta*, the large artery that takes blood away from the heart to the rest of the body. During systole, the aortic valve is open and blood flows freely to the rest of your body.

- ✔ The second number is the *diastolic blood pressure* (DBP), the lowest point of blood pressure. After your heart empties the blood from the ventricle, the aortic valve shuts to prevent blood from returning into the heart from the rest of your body. Your heart muscle relaxes and the ventricle expands as blood from the lungs fills it up. At that moment, the blood pressure rapidly falls within your arteries until it reaches its DBP, its lowest point. Before the pressure falls further, the ventricle contracts again and the blood pressure starts to rise back up to the systolic level.

With this information and the guidance in the following sections, you can determine whether your numbers are normal or high.

Clarifying what qualifies as "high blood pressure"

After you've established your SBP and DBP, your doctor determines whether your blood pressure is high and whether it should be treated. But first, how high is too high?

At birth, your blood pressure is around 90/60 mm Hg or even lower. It gradually rises as you grow older, and normal adult blood pressure is between 120/80 mm Hg and 139/89 mm Hg. Numbers higher than these indicate high blood pressure.

No fixed number serves as a guide for high diastolic or systolic blood pressure. Doctors have established 140/90 mm Hg as the point at which action is taken, but a person with a reading of 120/80 mm Hg is still at lower risk of blood pressure complications than a person with a 130/85 mm Hg.

Checking out the updated "Classification of Blood Pressure for Adults"

The National Heart, Lung, and Blood Institute (a division of the National Institutes of Health) established the Joint National Committee on Prevention, Detection, Evaluation, and Treatment of High Blood Pressure. The latest incarnation of the committee, *JNC 7,* published its data in 2003 and rewrote the Classification of Blood Pressure for Adults. Table 2-1 shows this latest classification. Use the table to determine whether your blood pressure measurement is normal or abnormal. If your blood pressure falls in the prehypertension or high blood pressure categories, discuss treatment with your doctor. (Refer to Part III of this book for information on successful treatment options.) *Note:* When SBP and DBP fall into two different categories, use the higher one.

Table 2-1	Classification of Blood Pressure for Adults*		
Category	*SBP (mm Hg)*		*DBP (mm Hg)*
Normal	<120	And	<80
Prehypertension	120–139	Or	80–89
Stage 1 HBP	140–159	Or	90–99
Stage 2 HBP	>160	Or	>100

*As noted by the Joint National Committee on Prevention, Detection, Evaluation, and Treatment of High Blood Pressure.

This new classification recognizes that the relationship between heart disease and blood pressure is continuous. Disease does not suddenly start at a blood pressure of 140/90. The higher the blood pressure, the greater the risk of a heart attack, heart failure, brain attack, or kidney failure. JNC 7 found that for adults 40 to 70 years of age, each increase of systolic blood pressure of 20 mm Hg or diastolic blood pressure of 10 mm Hg above 115/75 doubles the risk of one of those complications.

JNC 7 introduced the concept of *prehypertension* to emphasize that even a blood pressure of 120/80 can have medical consequences and needs to be addressed. One in five Americans has prehypertension. If you're in this category, the risk that you'll develop complications of high blood pressure is greater than if your blood pressure were in the normal range. You need to make lifestyle changes to get the readings down to the normal level. (I discuss these changes in detail in Chapters 9, 10, 11 and 12.)

When JNC 7 created the prehypertension classification, 50 million Americans who thought they had normal blood pressure suddenly found themselves in a new category that required treatment. Some skeptical people suggested that the drug industry benefited the most from this change because a certain number of these people with prehypertension will end up on drugs. Actually, the government guidelines don't recommend drug treatment for prehypertension *unless* the meds are required for another condition like diabetes or chronic kidney disease. However, so many people fit into this category that many of them will inevitably receive drug treatment.

Perhaps the term *prehypertension* is an unfortunate one. It suggests that you are going to have a problem but don't have one yet. The truth is that making healthy changes in the prehypertensive state may help to avoid the even worse consequences of the hypertensive state. Lowering blood pressure by a few millimeters of mercury within this prehypertensive range has been shown to reduce sickness and death associated with high blood pressure. A better term may be *early hypertension* or *lower-risk hypertension*. These terms emphasize that the risk is not as great, but it exists.

You can't see or feel prehypertension. You must have your blood pressure measured as I describe earlier in this chapter.

Lowering Blood Pressure Too Much

People can tolerate many different levels of blood pressure without symptoms. But blood pressure can certainly be too low in a number of situations (for example, when a person takes too much blood-pressure-lowering medication, has diabetes, requires prolonged bed rest, or experiences bleeding or dehydration). Such patients discover how to get up slowly to give the body a chance to adjust. If the pressure is too low, the patient becomes dizzy upon standing because too much blood pools in the legs. In these cases, some kind of treatment is needed to raise the blood pressure.

Besides the drugs that treat high blood pressure, medications that may cause too-low blood pressure include

- Alcohol
- Antidepressants
- Heart medications
- Medications to treat anxiety
- Narcotic pain killers
- Prostate medications

Many medical conditions can also cause too-low blood pressure. Among them are

- Changes in heart rhythm
- Heart attack
- Heart failure (see Chapter 5)
- Severe allergic reactions

Some people's blood pressure actually lowers too much during sleep. The insufficient blood flow may increase the risk for heart attacks and brain attacks, and the fall may be even worse when a person takes blood-pressure-lowering drugs. At the present time, doctors have few solutions for this problem; the only treatment is to keep the amount of drugs at a level that doesn't worsen the condition.

Recognizing the White Coat Effect and Other Causes of Variable Readings

Blood pressure varies widely. If you check the blood pressure of a group of people at many different times of day or night, you find some amazing variations. For example, one person's blood pressure during the day can vary from 175/100 mm Hg (a high blood pressure) to 105/60 mm Hg, a healthy, normal blood pressure. Some of the reasons for the variability are

✔ Blood pressure tends to drop during sleep.

✔ Blood pressure quickly increases when you awaken.

✔ Respiration and heart rate affect blood pressure.

✔ Mental and physical activity affect blood pressure.

✔ The nighttime fall in blood pressure is less in the elderly or people with diabetes.

✔ Smoking raises blood pressure with each cigarette.

✔ Sleep deprivation raises blood pressure.

✔ Defecation or a bladder full of urine may raise blood pressure.

✔ Consuming more than two ounces of alcohol on a daily basis raises blood pressure.

Another factor that often causes a rise in blood pressure is the *white coat effect,* which means something about physicians frightens a patient, causing the patient's systolic blood pressure to be 10 millimeters of mercury higher when the physician takes it as compared to when the nurse takes it. ***Note:*** Even the nurse can cause a mild white coat effect. If you take your blood pressure at home, it may be another 5 millimeters or so lower than the nurse's reading.

Interestingly, the same physician gets an even higher reading when he takes your blood pressure in the hospital than when he takes it in his office. If your physician gets a high reading, make sure he takes it again at least five minutes later in your visit; it often shows a dramatic fall, as much as 10 millimeters of mercury.

Eighty percent of patients who have high blood pressure in the doctor's office when measured correctly also have a high reading outside the office. The 20 percent who have normal blood pressure outside the office have the white coat effect.

Experiencing the white coat effect does not mean, however, that you're okay if your blood pressure is normal at home but not in the doctor's office. All the studies that show improvement in the rates of stroke, heart attacks, and other complications are based on measurements made in the doctor's office. People with white coat high blood pressure seem to be different from the population with normal blood pressure because those with the white coat effect often have associated health problems like high blood glucose and cholesterol. Their high blood pressure likely represents an abnormality consistent with their other abnormalities.

One way to get a definitive idea of whether you have high blood pressure is to have *ambulatory blood pressure monitoring* where you wear a device that measures your blood pressure for a day or two. If these measurements show high readings, you know your high blood pressure is real. I discuss the method later in this chapter.

Studies of the consequences of white coat high blood pressure are inconsistent. Some show increases in heart attacks and brain attacks; others fail to show this relationship. My advice is to use lifestyle changes to bring your blood pressure down (see Chapters 9, 10, 11, and 12 for details) and use medication only when you have other risk factors like diabetes or smoking. (Chapter 13 has full information about drug therapy.)

Taking Your Blood Pressure at Home

Often patients who register a high reading in the doctor's office register a normal reading at home. While normal home measurements don't mean that you can avoid treatment if your blood pressure is high in the doctor's office, a number of advantages exist to measuring your own blood pressure at home:

- ✔ You can identify whether you have white coat high blood pressure. (Refer to the previous section for more on this condition.)

- ✔ Frequent measurements of your blood pressure can tell you whether your treatment is working, and they can overcome the problem of blood pressure variability.

- ✔ You adhere to the treatment because you get rapid feedback.

- ✔ You know whether the diet, exercise, or pills are working, and you're able to alter the treatment long before your next office visit by getting in touch with your doctor by phone or e-mail.

- ✔ You may reduce the cost of care because you don't have to see your doctor as often if your blood pressure remains stable and low.

Because the home pressure tends to be lower, a normal pressure at home is less than 135/85 mm Hg.

Numerous devices are on the market for monitoring blood pressure at home. Some use the arm and some the wrist as the site of the measurement. I don't recommend using a mercury blood pressure gauge at home. Other types of blood pressure gauges are just as accurate and avoid the risk of mercury contamination.

The best home methods are electronic devices that measure the blood pressure at the elbow or wrist and only require you to attach the cuff properly and press a button. The device inflates the cuff, measures the blood pressure, and gives a reading on a screen. I have tested several of them in my office. Wrist and arm models by Panasonic and Omron are highly accurate, reliable, and should cost less than $100, which is a small price to pay for this level of quality. When you use the wrist models, remember to have your wrist at the level of your heart as you measure the blood pressure.

Even if you purchase one of these highly reliable home blood pressure monitoring devices, you must compare it with the results from a mercury blood pressure gauge at least once a year (every six months is even better) in your doctor's office. Accuracy is critical.

Obtaining an accurate blood pressure at home requires you to follow several rules. The most important ones are similar to blood pressure measurement in the doctor's office:

 ✔ Wait 15 minutes after exercising, eating, or drinking caffeine or alcohol.

 ✔ Rest five minutes before you take the measurement.

 ✔ Place your arm at the level of your heart.

 ✔ Be sure to record the reading with the date and time.

 ✔ Check your blood pressure in the morning and the evening.

Studies have shown that people who measure their own blood pressure are more likely to stay on a regimen for lowering their blood pressure. Purchase an accurate monitor that can remember your blood pressure readings, and download the numbers into a computer so your doctor can view them on his computer when you come to the office. You may avoid the need to take any medications!

Taking an Ambulatory Reading

An ambulatory reading uses a portable device called an *ambulatory blood pressure monitor* that consists of a cuff that attaches to your arm and to a machine. The machine pumps up the cuff and measures the blood pressure every 15 to 30 minutes during the day and every 30 to 60 minutes at night. Of course, the device is visible. The machine records the results and displays them when downloaded into a computer.

Your doctor may want to check your blood pressure many times during one 24-hour period for a variety of reasons. Some of them are

- To assess white coat high blood pressure (which I discuss earlier in this chapter)
- To determine whether you're resistant to drugs and, if so, why
- To check on low blood pressure symptoms
- To evaluate sporadic high blood pressure

Getting the Right Assessment

If, by chance, you're unable to prevent high blood pressure, make sure that your doctor evaluates your blood pressure properly. Assuming this is a first visit to the doctor for established high blood pressure, the doctor must make a number of assessments based on your history, a physical examination, and lab testing.

Assessing your history

Your history describes your past association with high blood pressure. It's similar to a history for any other condition but has a few variations specific to high blood pressure. The important points in the history are

- Duration of high blood pressure (when it was first discovered)
- Course of the blood pressure (whether it has always been high since it was discovered)
- Treatment with drugs, diet, exercise, or other means
- Use of agents that can worsen blood pressure such as steroids, birth control pills, and nonsteroidal anti-inflammatory agents
- Use of over-the-counter drugs such as decongestants or diet aids
- Any family history of high blood pressure
- Symptoms that may suggest secondary high blood pressure (see Chapter 4)
- Symptoms of the consequences of high blood pressure (see Part II)
- Presence of other risk factors like smoking, diabetes, high cholesterol, or kidney disease
- Social factors like family structure, work, and education
- Dietary history

✔ Sexual function (to evaluate before using drugs that affect it)

✔ Possibility of sleep *apnea* (when an individual gasps for breath and snores during sleep following several stops in breathing)

When patients are asked about symptoms before the diagnosis, they usually don't have any. But when they know they have high blood pressure, they tend to describe many symptoms including headache, ringing in the ears, dizziness, and fainting. In general, however, high blood pressure is not associated with symptoms.

Evaluating your physical exam

After the doctor notes the history, a physical examination follows. This is mostly a routine evaluation with some special studies because of the high blood pressure. The main parts of the exam are

✔ Abdominal exam to look for tumors or abnormal sounds suggesting restricted blood flow

✔ Blood pressure reading as I describe earlier in this chapter

✔ Evaluation of body fat distribution and waist circumference to look for *metabolic syndrome* (a condition often associated with high blood pressure where there is resistance to your own insulin)

✔ Examination of the neck for thyroid or blood vessel abnormalities

✔ Examination of the pulses in the arteries

✔ Heart exam

✔ Internal eye exam

✔ Lung exam

✔ Neurological exam

Using lab tests

Your history and physical exam can give the doctor an excellent idea of the severity of the problem and the possibility that secondary high blood pressure is present. Then lab tests provide a general picture of your overall health and look for specific abnormalities that the history and physical pointed to. The key lab tests for everyone with high blood pressure are

✔ Complete blood count

✔ Serum chemistry profile that looks at the sodium, potassium, glucose, liver function, and kidney function

✔ Lipid profile that evaluates cholesterol and triglycerides

✔ Microalbumin test to look for early kidney disease

After you have results for your total cholesterol, good cholesterol, and blood pressure, go to the following Web site for a prediction of your ten-year risk for a heart attack or death: `http://hp2010.nhlbihin.net/atpiii/ calculator.asp?usertype=pro`. The program also tells you how to interpret your individual risk. Based on that information, you know whether you need lifestyle modification with or without medication.

If the doctor suspects definite damage associated with high blood pressure, he should do other studies. For example:

✔ **Brain abnormalities:** A Doppler flow study checks for blockage of blood vessels in the neck.

✔ **Heart disease:** An electrocardiogram and chest X-ray check for heart damage.

✔ **Kidney problems:** An additional blood test checks for increased uric acid.

In Chapter 4, you can find the specific tests for secondary high blood pressure. Key elements in the history and physical that may lead a doctor to do these tests are

✔ The sudden onset of high blood pressure, especially under the age of 20 or above the age of 50

✔ Especially high blood pressure

✔ A low potassium level or a poor response to treatment

Use these preceding guidelines to determine whether your doctor is doing everything necessary to evaluate your high blood pressure. You may find that an element has been left out. Don't hesitate to inform the doctor and get the study. It's a matter of your health and your life.

Chapter 3

...ining Whether ...'re at Risk

● ●

...gh blood pressure

...'t do to bring down high blood pressure

● ●

...role in the development of high blood pressure. ...'t control some (like your family history, ethnic background, age, and gender), you can control others such as diet, exercise, stress, your smoking and drinking habits, and a tendency to park as close to the exercise facility as possible. Each factor may be present to a greater or lesser extent in a particular area of the world, so the prevalence of high blood pressure is low in some places and extremely high with severe consequences in other places (see Part II).

In this chapter, I discuss both the uncontrollable and the controllable factors related to the development of high blood pressure. If you haven't been diagnosed with high blood pressure, be sure to read up on the controllable factors that can help lessen your chances of developing it. If you have been diagnosed with high blood pressure, be sure to read Part III, where I discuss the same controllable factors in relation to treating high blood pressure.

Note: One factor that causes your blood pressure to rise is forgetting your spouse's birthday. Running over your son's bike when you back into the garage is another. Fortunately for you, the rise from this kind of event is only temporary!

The various factors leading to high blood pressure that I mention in this chapter are far from inclusive. I stress the most important ones, but scientists are continually discovering other factors that cause high blood pressure. If you want to discover more about the latest research, check out the appendix for updated references.

Clarifying What You Can't Control

This section describes the factors in your life that you can't control. You can't alter your family history, ethnic background, gender, and age. ***Note:*** These uncontrollable factors aren't quite the same as when you let a shirt hang in your closet for a while and it shrinks two sizes!

Although you can't control some factors, you still need to know how they contribute to high blood pressure, and you need to be cautious. Allow yourself to become obese, and you may have high blood pressure even though you're in a low-risk group.

Looking at the global picture

The prevalence of high blood pressure throughout the world breaks down into four major categories as follows:

- **Zero:** A few isolated groups such as those in the Amazon have zero high blood pressure.

- **Low:** The incidence of high blood pressure is low (below 15 percent) in the rural populations of Latin and South America, China, and Africa.

- **Normal:** Most often, high blood pressure prevails in 15 to 30 percent of a given population including most industrialized areas — Japan, Europe, and the Caucasian population of the United States.

- **High:** A high percentage (30 to 40 percent) exists in the Russian Federation, Finland, Poland, and among African Americans.

Wherever high blood pressure occurs, heart, brain, and kidney complications (see Part II) are similarly high. The burden of disease due to high blood pressure is enormous in countries like the Russian Federation, but no more than among African Americans. (See the "African Americans" section later in this chapter.) Brain attack, usually related to high blood pressure, is the second leading cause of death in Japan, and researchers continue to emphasize the control of blood pressure to prevent strokes (*Stroke,* August 2001).

Several studies conducted throughout the world on high blood pressure show that a high percentage of high blood pressure often coexists with poor awareness and insufficient treatment. For example:

- A study in the *Archives of Brazilian Cardiology* (July 2001) shows that the percentages of high blood pressure in Brazil are similar to the United States' numbers, but because of a combination of poor awareness and poor treatment, only a fraction of that Brazilian population can control it.

✔ Several European populations are aware of their high blood pressure but are unable to control it. For example:

- In Spain, a blood pressure of 160/95 mm Hg (rather than the 140/90 mm Hg recommended by JNC 7; see Chapter 2) is the cutoff point to begin treatment.

- In France, both awareness and treatment are inadequate.

✔ Although many South Koreans have high blood pressure and receive treatment, few South Koreans are able to control their high blood pressure according to a study in the *Journal of Hypertension* (September 2001).

Before you pack your bags and fly off to the Amazon in hopes of living a long, illness-free retirement in a tropical paradise, please consider this possibility: If a high percentage of high blood pressure often coexists with poor awareness and insufficient treatment, then *perhaps* low percentages can coexist with acute awareness and sufficient treatment — without a trip to the Amazons! Read on.

Accounting for the contribution of your genes

High blood pressure tends to run in families, so a family history of the condition can predict its development in relatives who have normal blood pressure. For example, when comparing biological children with adopted children, the same or similar blood pressure measurements were shared between biological parents and their children to a greater degree than between adopted children and their parents. Bottom line? If you have two or more relatives who developed high blood pressure before the age of 55, you're at much higher risk of developing it yourself. (Next time around, try to pick your parents a little more carefully!)

Researchers still don't know exactly *how* and *which* genes are responsible for high blood pressure, but they do believe many genes contribute to the condition. In other words, having one particular gene doesn't predict high blood pressure — and even if they find the right ones, today's scientists can't alter genes.

Heredity also affects body weight. People who are closely related tend to have similar degrees of obesity, which plays a large role in the development of high blood pressure. (See the "Controlling your weight" section later in this chapter for more details about the effect of excess pounds.)

The Stroke Belt

The Stroke Belt includes most of the southeastern United States with the exception of Florida. The greater prevalence of high blood pressure in this area means that large numbers of strokes (brain attacks) occur there. In fact, deaths due to brain attacks in that area are more than 10 percent above the national average. But brain attacks aren't the only consequence of high blood pressure. Other complications such as kidney failure and heart failure occur far more often in the Southeast than throughout the rest of the country. (For more on brain attacks, kidney failure, and heart failure, see Part II.) In addition, the overall death rate is higher in the southeastern states as compared to the rest of the country.

Caucasian men in the Southeast have a somewhat higher prevalence of high blood pressure compared to the rest of the country. But low birth weight and high blood pressure are more frequent among African Americans in the Southeast, the area of the country where most African Americans live.

However, the reasons that African Americans in the southeastern United States have such high rates of high blood pressure and death due to its complications are no different from the reasons for high blood pressure in general:

✔ **High salt intake** is common in the Southeast, especially among African Americans.

✔ **Low potassium intake** from fruits and vegetables is usual.

✔ **Obesity** occurs in a much greater percentage of the population.

✔ **Physical inactivity** is the rule in the Southeast. Half of the population doesn't get enough exercise.

The *insulin resistance syndrome* may be a particularly important example of the role that inheritance plays in high blood pressure. People with this condition have

✔ Increased *insulin* (the hormone that controls blood sugar) and at the same time reduced sensitivity to their insulin

✔ A typical pattern of blood fats consisting of high triglycerides (the type of fat on meat — greater than 200 mg/dL) and low HDL cholesterol (the blood fat particle that protects against heart attacks — less than 30 mg/dL)

In addition, people who suffer from insulin resistance syndrome

✔ Are usually but not always obese

✔ Tend to have a much higher incidence of fatal heart attacks

✔ May make up 20 percent of all high blood pressure cases

✔ Tend to carry their fat around the waistline

Estimating the effects of ethnicity

According to the United States Centers for Disease Control and Prevention, the prevalence of high blood pressure was reduced among men and women in every ethnic group between 1960 and 1990, but then the prevalence increased between 1990 and 2002 (the last year for which data is available). Some representative differences are shown in Table 3-1.

Table 3-1	Percentage of United States Population Age 20 and Older with High Blood Pressure*				
Group	*1960*	*1970*	*1980*	*1990*	*2002*
Both sexes	36.9	38.3	39.0	23.1	33.6
Male	40.0	42.4	44.0	25.3	30.6
Female	33.7	34.4	34.0	20.8	31.0
Caucasian Male	39.3	41.7	43.5	24.3	32.5
Caucasian Female	31.7	32.4	32.3	19.3	31.9
African American Male	48.1	51.8	48.7	34.9	42.6
African American Female	50.8	50.3	47.5	33.8	46.6
Hispanic Male			25.0	25.2	26.3
Hispanic Female			21.8	22.0	23.4

Percentages provided by the U.S. Centers for Disease Control and Prevention.

The table shows the great strides that have been made to reduce the prevalence of high blood pressure in this 42-year period. But the table indicates that nearly a third of the age-20-and-older population suffers from high blood pressure and two out of five African Americans have high blood pressure. When coupled with appropriate medical attention and lifestyle changes (which I describe later in this chapter), awareness of these factors can lower the number of high blood pressure cases in the United States.

African Americans

African Americans — the population most at risk in the United States for developing high blood pressure and its consequences — develop high blood pressure twice as often as Caucasians. In addition, African Americans

✔ Have a high rate of *end-stage renal disease* (kidney failure), which may be due in part to their increased level of high blood pressure

✔ May have an inherited kidney defect that limits their ability to handle salt

✔ Have a lower response to nitric oxide (a necessary compound in the blood vessels) than Caucasians (For more on nitric oxide, see the nearby "Nitric oxide to the rescue" sidebar.)

In addition, the stresses associated with low socioeconomic status are frequently blamed for at least some of the high blood pressure among African Americans.

Dietary treatment, however, has been particularly successful among African Americans with high blood pressure. One of the best approaches has been the Dietary Approach to Stop Hypertension (DASH diet — see Chapter 9), which consists of increased amounts of fruits, vegetables, grains, low-fat dairy products, and low-fat protein.

Hispanics

The prevalence of high blood pressure among Hispanics is generally similar to Caucasians. Although the incidence of high blood pressure is greater among African Americans, Hispanic adults tend not to take medication for their high blood pressure as often as Caucasians or African Americans.

Caucasians

About 30 percent of adult Caucasians in the United States have high blood pressure. Caucasians, as a group, seem to be more aware of their high blood pressure and get treatment more often than African Americans or Hispanics. However, Caucasians' treatment is satisfactory only about 20 percent of the time, so they also have much room for improvement; in this case, the problem is often due to a lack of patient compliance with the medication.

Nitric oxide to the rescue

The cells that line the inside of the blood vessels produce *nitric oxide,* a potent compound that widens blood vessels and reduces blood pressure. A number of risk factors for cardiovascular disease cause damage to these cells and inhibit their ability to produce nitric oxide. These risk factors include

✔ High blood pressure

✔ High cholesterol

✔ Insulin resistance

✔ Postmenopausal lack of estrogen

✔ Tobacco smoking or chewing

When these risk factors are present, they also make the individual more susceptible to the blood-pressure-raising effect of stress. Reversing these risk factors eliminates their damaging effects and helps restore nitric oxide production. Part III explains ways to attack any of these risk factors.

Identifying the culprits: Salt and fat

By comparing people of the same race in different areas of the world, a 1999 study in *Scientific American* sought an explanation for the high rate of high blood pressure among African Americans. The authors, dissatisfied with a genetic explanation, found great differences between Africans living in Nigeria, Jamaica, and the United States:

✔ Nigerians are generally lean, do physically demanding work, and eat a traditional Nigerian diet of rice, vegetables, and fruits. Blood pressure doesn't rise as they get older, and high blood pressure is rare.

✔ The Jamaican diet is a mixture of home-grown and commercial foods. They tend to live six years longer than African Americans because the incidence of cancer and heart disease is lower.

✔ In Maywood, Illinois, an African American community just outside of Chicago, the migrants from the southeastern United States have a high-salt, high-fat diet.

Although all the groups had a common genetic background, the percentage of the population with high blood pressure was 7 percent for the Nigerians, 26 percent for the Jamaicans, and 33 percent for the African Americans. The Americans also had greater body weight, greater salt intake, and less potassium intake than Nigerians.

The authors concluded that no racial explanation exists. High blood pressure in African Americans isn't genetic because African Americans with high blood pressure and those with normal blood pressure share the same genes. The study emphasizes that explanations for the various results should be sought in the environment and not in the genes. The Nigerians ate less salt, consumed more potassium, and were much more physically active.

Focusing on gender

Boys are much more likely than girls to have higher systolic blood pressure (the amount of pressure in your arteries as the heart pumps; see Chapter 2 for more details). In a study in the December 2006 *Circulation,* starting at age 12 and every two years thereafter, high blood pressure increased 19 percent in boys but was stable for girls in Canada. The key factors were a sedentary lifestyle and lack of exercise in both boys and girls. I say a lot more about high blood pressure and children in Chapter 15.

In young adults (ages 18 to 35), high blood pressure is more prevalent in men than women. But after women reach the age of 50 (when most women lose their estrogen through menopause or removal of their ovaries), women have a higher prevalence of high blood pressure than men.

However, more often than men, women tend to be aware of their high blood pressure, get treatment for it, and control it. The explanation for this difference may be that women see doctors more frequently due to pregnancies, pelvic exams, and breast exams — all opportunities for the doctor to note high blood pressure.

Similar to men, women reduce their risk of brain attack when treated for high blood pressure, so treatment should be given to women just as often as it's given to men.

In the following sections, I describe the effects of oral contraceptives and menopause on women's blood pressure.

Taking oral contraceptives

Previously, oral contraceptives contained more estrogen and progesterone than they do today, and their use was associated with more heart disease, heart attacks, brain attacks, and a higher death rate. Current preparations contain less hormone and do not cause those complications, especially in comparison to other methods of contraception. However, oral contraceptives can cause a slight increase in blood clots and breast cancer, so a woman who has had blood clots in the past should not take oral contraceptives.

Oral contraceptives are associated with some rise in blood pressure, which subsides when the contraceptive is discontinued. However, once in a while, oral contraceptives can bring on more severe high blood pressure. If a patient has a family history of high blood pressure or kidney disease, the physician needs to be cautious about giving her oral contraceptives and then monitor her blood pressure frequently.

Exactly why blood pressure rises as a result of taking oral contraceptives is unclear, but the amount of progesterone (not estrogen) in the preparation may be the problem. Preparations that contain less progesterone or intermittent progesterone are less often connected to high blood pressure in the patient.

If the blood pressure doesn't return to normal when a woman discontinues the oral contraceptive, she should be evaluated for some other cause. A woman who can't use another form of contraception may need to combine the oral contraceptive with a blood-pressure-lowering drug. (See Chapter 13 for more information on pressure-lowering medications.)

Going past menopause

Unlike women who have not yet reached menopause, postmenopausal women — even those who have normal blood pressure — respond to stress with a rise in their blood pressure. The estrogen loss that occurs during menopause may not be the only factor; the weight gain that accompanies aging and other factors like diminished exercise may also contribute to the rise. *Note:* Postmenopausal women are actually more sensitive to salt than men are, and this sensitivity may be an additional reason for their increased tendency towards high blood pressure.

Taking estrogenic hormones doesn't seem to elevate blood pressure or make the postmenopausal woman more sensitive to salt or stress. For this reason, postmenopausal women who have high blood pressure may be given estrogens.

Rising in stages with age

Blood pressure tends to go up with age for many reasons — reduction in kidney function, less ability to rid the body of salt, hardening of the arteries, increasing obesity, and greater sensitivity to salt's blood-pressure-raising effect.

With aging, the blood pressure tends to rise in stages. Although these stages vary for some individuals, high blood pressure usually develops in a fairly orderly fashion — from pre-high blood pressure to sustained high blood pressure.

High blood pressure can occur before age 30, but the usual sequence of events is as follows:

✔ **Between birth and the age of 30 (pre-high blood pressure stage):** Occasional blood pressure measurements may be high, but the elevation isn't constant. However, even an occasional rise is a clue that high blood pressure may develop. Other clues are

- Birth weight is low.

- Blood pressure rises excessively during stress or exercise.

- Random pressure checks are high/normal (close to 140/90 mm Hg).

- Other features such as obesity, increased alcohol intake, diabetes, reduced HDL cholesterol, or increased triglycerides may be present.

✔ **Usually between the ages of 30 and 40:** This stage may last five to ten years. High blood pressure occurs frequently, but periods of normal blood pressure follow.

✔ **As early as 30 years of age, but usually by the age of 50 (*essential hypertension* — sustained high blood pressure for which the cause cannot be determined):** People who suffer from essential hypertension at age 50 or sooner are highly susceptible to early heart attacks and brain attacks. If left untreated, their life expectancy is reduced 15 to 20 years.

✔ **Past the age of 50:** This condition is more likely to be *secondary* (from other causes) high blood pressure, as I explain in Chapter 4. Chapter 14 discusses the problems of blood pressure in the elderly at greater length.

Preventing High Blood Pressure with Lifestyle Changes

Every year, 2 million new patients are diagnosed with high blood pressure every year in the United States. Although you can't change the genes that you received from your parents, you can change many lifestyle behaviors to prevent high blood pressure. For starters, all adults should be screened for high blood pressure at least every two years. Other changes you can make include

- ✔ Reducing your stress using humor (see Chapter 8)

- ✔ Increasing your potassium intake by eating more fruits and vegetables (see Chapter 9)

- ✔ Reducing daily salt intake to less than 6,000 milligrams (1 teaspoon), which is equal to 2,400 milligrams of sodium (see Chapter 10)

- ✔ Keeping alcohol intake to two drinks or less per day (see Chapter 11)

- ✔ Controlling your weight through diet (see Chapter 9) and exercise (see Chapter 12)

All the techniques that *prevent* high blood pressure can also help *lower* blood pressure after it is present. But the greatest differences between prevention and treatment are the costs and risks of the medication that most people need to treat their high blood pressure. If you can prevent high blood pressure, do everything in your power to do so. You won't be sorry.

Reducing tension

Essential high blood pressure (see the previous section "Rising in stages with age") is due equally to inheritance and the environment. The major factors in the environment are diet and psychological and social stresses.

Many groups show the effects of stressful situations on blood pressure. For example:

- ✔ A study in the *New England Journal of Medicine* (March 1968) compared several nuns isolated in Italy to a group of women in regular society. Blood pressures were the same at the beginning, but after 30 years, the nuns' blood pressures were 30 millimeters lower than the other group's.

- ✔ People who go from low-stress societies (like the Nigerians in Africa that I describe in the previous section) to higher-stress societies (like Africans in America) show sustained increases in blood pressure.

- People who work in jobs where they have little control but much responsibility show elevated blood pressures.

- Air traffic controllers have higher blood pressures as a group than people in less stressful occupations.

- African Americans growing up in higher-stress environments have a higher incidence of high blood pressure.

Some of these studies have been questioned because of other contributing factors. For example, the diet of the nuns may have been less likely to cause high blood pressure, especially over 30 years. People going to higher-stress societies are also eating more salt than they did before.

Although some studies show a correlation between internalized anger, other studies don't. Whether blood pressure tends to be high in certain individuals who turn their anger inward rather than responding by an external show of anger or some other external act (like increased exercise) is still the subject of much controversy.

Finally, do people who respond to stress by reacting excessively tend to develop high blood pressure more often than people who are less reactive? The answer isn't clear; studies of this phenomenon are again inconsistent.

Many studies on stress and high blood pressure result in inconsistent findings, but one fact is certain: Reducing the level of stress in your life can only do you good. The less stressed you are, the less likely you are to overeat, smoke, and drink excessively — all factors known to cause high blood pressure. Chapter 8 introduces you to one great form of stress reduction — laughter.

Controlling your weight

The significance of an inactive lifestyle in the development of high blood pressure is clear. In study after study, people who exercise more have a lower incidence of high blood pressure, and active lifestyles promote weight control.

For every 10-pound weight gain, the systolic blood pressure goes up 4 to 5 millimeters of mercury. Therefore, you don't have to be overweight or obese for weight gain to raise your blood pressure.

Central obesity (fat in the waist area) is associated with high blood pressure more than obesity in the legs and thighs. A large waistline is a good clue that high blood pressure is on its way or has already arrived.

The insulin resistance syndrome (I describe this condition earlier in the "Accounting for the contribution of your genes" section) contains factors that place the patient at high risk of heart disease:

- Obesity
- High blood pressure
- Elevated levels of insulin and insulin resistance
- Central distribution of fat
- High triglycerides
- Low HDL (*good* cholesterol) and higher levels of LDL (*bad* cholesterol)
- High levels of uric acid in the bloodstream
- *Type 2 diabetes mellitus* (formerly called *non-insulin-dependent diabetes*)
- High levels of chemicals that prevent clots from breaking down

Just how obesity results in higher blood pressure is unclear. But scientists do know the following:

- People who are obese have increased *cardiac output* (flow of blood from the heart) and increased *peripheral resistance* (resistance to the passage of blood through the arteries). As a result, more blood needs to be pumped to provide nutrients to their bodies' increased tissues.
- Many organs, particularly the kidneys, don't accept increased blood flow, so they produce hormones to reduce it by narrowing the arteries, thus increasing peripheral resistance and blood pressure.
- Obese people often take in more salt than lean people, and they're more sensitive to the blood-pressure-raising effect of salt.
- Obesity is associated with an increase in the activity of the nervous system, which can cause narrowing of blood vessels.

In Chapter 9, I recommend weight loss as one treatment of high blood pressure. Combined with exercise (which I discuss in Chapter 12) and salt and alcohol reduction, weight loss can have a profound blood-pressure-lowering effect. **Note:** These measures should always precede pressure-lowering medications unless the blood pressure is dangerously high (greater than 180/120 mm Hg). Part of the positive effects of these lifestyle changes may include improvement in the insulin resistance syndrome, leading to reduced insulin and its role in raising blood pressure.

Of course, you don't want to take this exercise program too far. My grandmother started walking 5 miles a day at age 60. She's 97 now, and nobody knows where the heck she is!

Using less salt

The typical diet throughout the wealthier nations of the world contains too much salt. Evidence abounds. Not all people, however, develop high blood pressure; only about half the population. So, people who have high blood pressure must have some form of increased *sensitivity* (salt raises their blood pressure to a greater extent). The evidence for the role of salt comes from population studies as well as experimental manipulation of salt intake. The population studies noted that

- ✔ Primitive tribes that don't eat salt have zero high blood pressure; they also don't have the consequences of high blood pressure — damage to the heart, kidney, or brain.
- ✔ When these same primitive people eat salt, they develop high blood pressure and its consequences.
- ✔ The more salt consumed, the higher the blood pressure.

Experimental studies concluded that

- ✔ When people with high blood pressure restrict their salt, they lower their blood pressure.
- ✔ Babies with a low-salt diet have lower blood pressures.
- ✔ Animals that consume more salt show a rise in blood pressure.

This sensitivity to salt seems to be inherited from the mother because she usually has the same rise in blood pressure as her offspring after eating salt. A person without salt sensitivity excretes most excess salt along with water in the kidneys, but a person with salt sensitivity can't do this as easily.

Blood pressure, however, doesn't always fall when salt is restricted because certain groups of people are more salt sensitive. These include

- ✔ Diabetics
- ✔ Older individuals
- ✔ People whose kidneys are failing
- ✔ People who don't produce enough *renin,* an enzyme that raises blood pressure in their kidneys

Lowering your salt intake can help reduce your chances of developing high blood pressure. Paying attention to product labels and choosing foods labeled *sodium-free* or *reduced-sodium* can help you monitor your salt intake. I detail other practical ways to reduce your salt intake in Chapter 10.

Cutting out smoking and excessive drinking

Using tobacco in any form and drinking excessively (see Chapter 11) raise blood pressure, while the absence of smoking and drinking lowers blood pressure. Although tobacco and alcohol cause all kinds of other problems for you, their effect on your blood pressure is enough reason to stop using them.

Chapter 4

Dealing with Secondary High Blood Pressure

*S*econdary high blood pressure means that a specific disease causes the high blood pressure — the high blood pressure is one of several signs and symptoms associated with the disease. If the person is cured of the disease that's causing the secondary high blood pressure, then the high blood pressure is lowered. Treatment of the disease often eliminates the high blood pressure.

Although secondary high blood pressure makes up only 5 percent of the total number of high-blood-pressure cases, its causes are important. A careful history, physical exam, and lab evaluation (as I discuss in Chapter 2) can help a physician discover the disease that's causing your blood pressure to rise. This chapter introduces you to some of the most common causes of secondary high blood pressure, the way the diagnosis is confirmed in each case, and the appropriate treatment.

As you read the disease descriptions, you may imagine that you indeed have one of them. But chances are, you're more likely to win the lottery or be hit by a bolt of lightning than contract any one of these rare diseases. Of course, if you do get one, you'll be the only one on your block. (I recommend that you express your uniqueness some other way!)

The upside of secondary high blood pressure is that after you're treated for the primary disease, you're like new — most of the time. The high blood pressure and other signs and symptoms of the disease disappear. Your whole life improves — even your piano playing (if you then take lessons).

So before you let your imagination run wild about having one of these diseases, ask your doctor. If your doctor's opinion doesn't satisfy you, then get a second opinion from another physician.

Treating the disease or disorder that's causing the secondary high blood pressure can lower your blood pressure, but lifestyle changes can also lower secondary high blood pressure independent of the disease or disorder. This means that weight loss (see Chapter 9), exercise (see Chapter 12), stopping smoking (see Chapter 11), and reducing salt in your diet (see Chapter 10) can all make a big difference.

Finding Secondary High Blood Pressure Early

Several clues that should prompt an investigation for secondary high blood pressure include the following:

- Damage to the eyes, kidneys, or heart
- Family history of kidney disease
- Flushing spells (when your skin turns red and hot)
- Increased body pigmentation and pigmented stretch marks
- Intolerance to heat
- Loud humming sound in the abdomen (called a *bruit*)
- Low potassium level in the blood
- Poor response to usually effective treatment for high blood pressure
- Rapid pulse
- The onset of high blood pressure before age 20 or past age 50
- Unusually high blood pressure (above 180/120 mm Hg)

If you have any condition in the preceding list, point it out to your doctor. By finding and treating secondary high blood pressure early, you're more certain to return to normal before permanent changes occur. Some changes such as kidney damage can affect your high blood pressure permanently even when the primary disease or disorder is eliminated.

Evaluating the Role of Your Kidneys in Secondary High Blood Pressure

When high blood pressure is present, the kidneys always get involved. If the high blood pressure precedes the kidney damage, the high blood pressure is *primary* or *essential*. But when damage to the kidneys occurs first, then the high blood pressure is *secondary*. Two main conditions of the kidney — damaged kidney tissue and blocked kidney arteries — can lead to high blood pressure.

Certain drugs (particularly phenacetin, acetaminophen, and the nonsteroidal anti-inflammatory agents) can cause impaired kidney function. They're associated with wasting salt instead of retaining it though, so high blood pressure isn't usually the problem. And despite the loss of an entire kidney, a person who donates a kidney doesn't necessarily develop high blood pressure.

Discovering damaged kidney tissue

Damaged kidney tissue is the most common reason for secondary high blood pressure, accounting for about 50 percent of the cases. *Renal* (kidney) *parenchymal* (tissue) *hypertension* (high blood pressure) results from:

- A kidney-damaging illness such as diabetes
- Use of certain medications (see the *Tip* in the intro to this section)
- An inflammation of the kidney
- An injury to the kidney
- A hereditary disease that results in *cysts* (sacs filled with fluid)

The damaged kidneys don't function normally and can't eliminate sodium at a normal rate, resulting in salt and water retention that leads to high blood pressure.

Diagnosing chronic and acute kidney tissue damage

Loss of kidney tissue that leads to high blood pressure can be *chronic* (slow to develop) or *acute* (sudden). Some of the diseases and conditions that cause chronic kidney damage are

- Chronic obstruction of the *ureter* (the tube that takes urine from the kidney to the bladder)
- Cysts that displace normal kidney tissue

- Damage to the *glomerulus* (the filtering part of the kidney)

- *Diabetes mellitus* (diabetic kidney disease; see the nearby sidebar "The details of diabetic kidney disease" for more information)

The resulting secondary high blood pressure must be controlled because it can damage the kidneys further and lead to even higher blood pressure. It's a vicious cycle.

High blood pressure also accompanies *acute* kidney diseases (kidney diseases that occur in days, not weeks or months). Acute kidney disease isn't cute in any way; it's a sudden development of a lesion in the kidneys, and the person who develops it is usually pretty sick. Fortunately, it may go away just as rapidly as it develops. Two acute medical problems that can damage the kidneys are the following:

- ***Acute glomerulonephritis*** is seen in children and adults who suddenly pass dark urine and have swelling of the face. Its name comes from the inflammation that affects the kidney's *glomeruli,* the structures that filter the blood. The disease can occur after a sore throat caused by a bacteria called *streptococcus.* The blood pressure rises during the time the patient is ill and is treated with salt restriction and drugs if necessary.

- ***Ureteral obstruction*** occurs when a compression from a tumor or other tissue closes the tubes that carry urine to the bladder. For example, a tumor of the prostate gland can cause the compression. The blockage may be on one kidney or both. Relieving the obstruction usually relieves the high blood pressure.

These two sources of acute secondary high blood pressure are quite rare, representing less than 10 percent of cases involving the kidneys.

Other conditions that lead to acute kidney damage include blockage in the arteries to both kidneys, trauma to the kidneys, or certain X-ray or surgical procedures. For example, certain chemicals used to observe the kidneys during an X-ray may suddenly damage the kidneys, especially in people with diabetes. Surgery that accidentally damages the arteries to the kidneys also leads to a sudden rise in blood pressure. ***Note:*** Most acute kidney diseases resolve over time if the person receives the necessary medical support during the acute illness.

Testing for and treating damaged kidney tissue

Blood urea nitrogen (BUN) and *creatinine* are blood tests that can detect damage to the kidney by measuring products that are normally excreted in the urine. (When the kidneys are damaged, these waste products back up in the blood.) Unfortunately, these tests don't register abnormality until the latter stages of the disease, when more than half the kidney tissue is damaged.

The details of diabetic kidney disease

Diabetes mellitus, a particularly damaging disease that may affect the kidneys, is the most common cause of kidney damage and kidney failure. The disease usually takes 15 or more years of poorly controlled diabetes to affect the kidneys. Most people that have diabetes mellitus also have high blood pressure and *diabetic retinopathy,* the characteristic eye disease in diabetes. Certain drugs called *ACE inhibitors* (see Chapter 13) are particularly helpful in slowing the progression of diabetic kidney disease and may even reverse it.

In diabetic kidney disease, the most important treatments consist of controlling blood glucose (sugar), blood pressure, and blood cholesterol. Diabetics should restrict their salt intake as well as their protein, which seems to make the kidney disease worse.

Fortunately, a *microalbuminuria test,* which checks for *albumin* (a protein) seeping out of the kidney and into the urine, can signal kidney disease at an early stage — when protection of the kidneys and reversal of the disease are still possible. Checking the amount of protein in the urine can also be a useful test for the worsening of kidney disease because protein levels increase as kidneys lose more tissue.

A kidney *sonogram* is also useful for detecting kidney damage. The sonogram bounces sound off the kidney to evaluate its shape and size and to detect any kidney tissue loss.

If the various studies don't make the diagnosis, a kidney *biopsy* — the removal of tissue for diagnostic examination — can often give a definitive diagnosis.

When the disease has damaged the kidneys so severely that they can no longer perform their filtering function, the kidneys are in *end-stage renal disease* (also known as *kidney failure*). At this point, two treatment options exist (see Chapter 6 for more information on both options):

- ✔ **Dialysis (mechanically cleaning the blood of poisons):** During dialysis, high blood pressure is present and must be controlled. Reducing the amount of fluid in the body usually accomplishes this.

- ✔ **Kidney transplant:** High blood pressure can be a complication. Transplants are less of a problem when the healthy kidney comes from a person who doesn't have high blood pressure.

Handling blocked kidney arteries

Diseases that cause *renal* (kidney) *vascular* (blood vessel) *hypertension* (high blood pressure) block one or both kidney arteries. When the obstruction keeps a kidney from receiving enough blood flow, the kidney secretes *renin,* an enzyme that ultimately brings on high blood pressure. Because the original obstruction keeps the increased blood pressure from delivering more blood to the kidney, the high blood pressure continues.

The renin acts on *angiotensin I* (a hormone) to produce *angiotensin II,* a hormone that causes the contraction of blood vessels. Angiotensin II also stimulates the production of *aldosterone,* a hormone that causes salt and water retention. I discuss aldosterone in more detail later in this chapter.

Diagnosing blocked kidney arteries

Many diseases can cause obstruction of one or both of the kidney arteries. These diseases occur in about 6 out of 100,000 people and include

- **Atherosclerosis:** In this process, cholesterol is laid down in the arteries, eventually causing the arteries to narrow. This condition usually occurs in men over the age of 45 and it accounts for two-thirds of all blocked kidney arteries cases.

- **Fibromuscular disease:** The kidney artery and the body's arteries in general become thickened and narrowed, especially in young women under the age of 45 and in children who have the disease.

- **Aneurysms:** The kidney artery or the heart's *aorta* (the artery leading to the kidney's artery) can have a defect and balloon out, causing blockage. As a result, the normal passage for blood narrows and blood enters the wall of the artery. The great danger of aneurysms is bursting, which may lead to death through loss of blood.

- **Emboli-clots:** These blood clots block the artery.

A *bruit,* a humming sound in the abdomen, can signal these common causes of kidney artery obstruction. However, it can be heard in only 50 percent of the cases where a doctor listens with a stethoscope over the patient's abdomen.

Because the kidneys produce increased amounts of aldosterone when the kidney arteries are blocked, the potassium level decreases. So another warning sign is a low potassium level in the blood. This diagnosis is most often associated with high blood pressure (higher than 120 diastolic) that doesn't respond to treatment.

When a doctor suspects an artery-blocking disease, he can order a study of the arteries to the kidneys. As dye is injected into the kidney arteries, an X-ray displays the size of the arterial passage. This study can help with a diagnosis, but opening up the obstructed artery may not cure the high blood pressure if the disease has been going on for some time.

Treating blocked kidney arteries

At the time of the first edition of this book, enthusiasm for treating blocked kidney arteries with *angioplasty* (kidney artery expansion) was very high. During angioplasty, the surgeon inserts a *catheter* (a slender, hollow tube) into the artery and widens the artery with a balloon. Then he places a device called a *stent* in the artery to keep it open permanently.

None of the studies that showed such promise for angioplasty and stenting had *random controls* (to compare the outcome of a patient who received the angioplasty to a patient who received medical treatment). Such a study is taking place at the time of this writing, but the results won't be available for several years. Some of the issues that may make angioplasty less certain as the treatment of choice are

- ✔ Medical therapy with drugs is highly effective for many years in more than half the patients.

- ✔ Angioplasty fails to lower blood pressure in up to 40 percent of patients.

- ✔ Kidney function gets worse in at least 20 percent of patients treated with angioplasty.

- ✔ The disease recurs in up to 20 percent of patients who are initially successful, although the stent seems to increase the rate of success.

As a result of these findings, angioplasty is now delayed in many patients in favor of drugs, at least until kidney function begins to fall.

Because renin causes the increased blood pressure, an *angiotensin-converting enzyme (ACE) inhibitor* (a drug that blocks its effect; see the nearby sidebar "The details of diabetic kidney disease") can reverse the high blood pressure, but it may also reduce blood supply to the obstructed kidney. Patients who can't tolerate an ACE inhibitor because of the side effect of coughing do well with an *angiotensin II receptor blocker,* which does not produce a cough (see Chapter 13 for more about drug therapy).

Discovering Hormone-Secreting Tumors That Elevate Blood Pressure

Organs that normally make *hormones* (chemical messengers that trigger reactions) can develop tumors that also produce hormones. But the tumor's hormones elevate blood pressure to an abnormal extent. These tumors usually originate in an *adrenal gland* (one adrenal gland sits on top of each of your kidneys; see Figure 4-1) but can also arise in nerve tissues. The adrenal glands secrete the following hormones:

- ✓ **Epinephrine:** Maintains blood pressure and blood glucose
- ✓ **Aldosterone:** Controls salt and water levels in the bloodstream
- ✓ **Cortisol:** Maintains blood glucose (sugar) and also plays a role in maintaining blood pressure

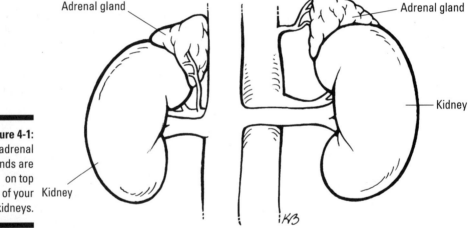

Adrenal gland

Adrenal gland

Kidney

Figure 4-1:
Your adrenal glands are on top of your kidneys.

Kidney

Figure 4-2 shows the different parts of the adrenal gland and the part responsible for the various hormones described in this section.

Finding an epinephrine-producing tumor

Epinephrine (adrenaline) and *norepinephrine,* normal products of the adrenal gland, raise blood pressure, heart rate, and blood glucose during stressful times and causes sweating. Sometimes a *pheochromocytoma* (a tumor that releases large quantities of norepinephrine) can arise in an adrenal gland (shown with the kidneys in Figure 4-1) or along many nerves.

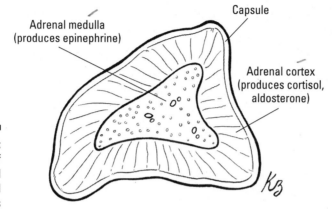

Adrenal medulla
(produces epinephrine)

Capsule

Adrenal cortex
(produces cortisol,
aldosterone)

Figure 4-2:
The parts of
the adrenal
gland
and its
hormones.

Diagnosing a pheochromocytoma

A pheochromocytoma is rare, arising in only 6 out of 100,000 people who have high blood pressure. However, the sudden release of a large amount of norepinephrine may be fatal.

WARNING!

A proper diagnosis is crucial because a pheochromocytoma can cause death if the patient experiences severe stress or trauma before the disease is discovered.

The most common, key symptoms of a pheochromocytoma are

- ✔ Headache
- ✔ *Palpitations* (the feeling that the heart is beating rapidly)
- ✔ Excessive sweating

Note: If high blood pressure is present but the patient feels none of these symptoms, the diagnosis of a pheochromocytoma is extremely unlikely. High blood pressure is sustained in over half the patients with this condition, but it may be intermittent.

Exercise, urination, defecation, an enema, smoking, examination of the abdomen, and anesthesia can bring on these attacks of headache, palpitations, and sweating, which can vary from severe to mild. The usual frequency is once a week, and the duration is less than one hour, but timing can be different for each patient.

Certain cheeses (especially aged cheddar and aged Stilton), beer, and wine that contain a chemical called *tyramine* may bring on a headache, palpitations, and sweating. Drugs like *histamine, glucagon,* and *phenothiazines* can also precipitate these symptoms.

A pheochromocytoma is suspected much more often than it actually occurs simply because its symptoms are the same as those of a healthy person who is nervous and upset.

The following steps explain how your doctor proceeds when she suspects a norepinephrine-producing tumor:

1. **A blood test for *metanephrine,* a breakdown product of epinephrine, screens for a pheochromocytoma.**

   Breakdown products result when epinephrine is converted to an inactive form in the body.

2. **If your metanephrine level is elevated, the doctor asks you to collect urine for 24 hours.**

   This test checks for the presence of metanephrine and *catecholamines* (other breakdown products of epinephrine).

3. **If elevated levels of metanephrine and catecholamines are found, a tumor can be located with a *computed tomography* (CT) or *magnetic resonance imaging* (MRI) scan (highly sensitive X-rays).**

   Most of these tumors locate in the adrenal gland, but 15 percent of them arise in another location such as the nerve tissue, the abdomen, or the chest cavity. (If the tumor is in one of these locations and is large enough, more than 2 centimeters, the scan can see it there as well). Nevertheless, the surgeon may have to find it during surgery, and usually the surgeon looks for more than the one tumor. About 10 percent of these tumors are malignant.

4. **If a CT or MRI scan doesn't identify a tumor, then you're injected with a radioactive substance, *metaiodobenzylguanidine* (MIBG).** (Try saying all that in one breath!)

   Because pheochromocytomas absorb MIBG, a radiation counter passed over the body can detect the excessive radiation in a particular area to locate the tumor.

Forms of pheochromocytoma run in families as solitary pheochromocytoma or along with other tumors. When several different types of tumors are present, the condition is *multiple endocrine neoplasia* and involves other glands. The doctor should look for tumors specifically of the thyroid and parathyroid glands whenever a pheochromocytoma is discovered.

(as ling nglio)

If I suspected that I had a pheochromocytoma (given the fact that I, like the vast majority of doctors, much less endocrinologists, have never seen a case after 30 years of practice), I would get on the next plane to one of the centers that has some significant experience with this condition: the Mayo Clinic, the Cleveland Clinic, or the National Institutes of Health.

Treating a pheochromocytoma

Surgery removes most pheochromocytomas, but first the patient's blood pressure has to be under control. The doctor may prescribe *dibenzyline* to block the action of epinephrine and control the high blood pressure. A week of dibenzyline or *doxazosin,* a similar drug, is sufficient, but a patient with severely high blood pressure may need injections of *phentolamine* in the vein every five minutes until the blood pressure is controlled so surgery can proceed.

If the blood pressure isn't controlled before this surgery, the death rate can be as high as 50 percent. However, the likelihood of the blood pressure not being controlled first is extremely rare.

The surgery is *laparoscopic* (minimally invasive removal of the tumor through a small incision in the abdomen). A tube is inserted, and the tumor is localized and removed. (Believe me, it's not as easy as it sounds. You should watch at least a couple before trying it!) This surgery can be done on an outpatient basis, and two weeks later the patient can return to normal activity. By comparison, the old technique of conventional surgery required five to seven days in the hospital and a four-week recovery period.

Like with other secondary causes of high blood pressure, the high blood pressure may persist after surgery if permanent changes have occurred. The patient then needs blood pressure pills (see Chapter 13 for more about drug therapy).

Detecting a tumor that produces aldosterone

The *adrenal cortex* (the outer covering of the adrenal gland; refer to Figure 4-2) secretes aldosterone, an important hormone that's responsible for retaining salt and eliminating potassium from the body. *Primary hyperaldosteronism* (a malfunction usually due to an aldosterone-producing tumor in one of the adrenal glands) may produce an overabundance of aldosterone — more than the human body can safely handle. The large amount of aldosterone causes significant sodium retention, potassium loss, and high blood pressure.

Similar to the prevalence of pheochromocytoma (see the "Diagnosing a pheochromocytoma" section earlier in this chapter), the incidence of aldosterone-producing tumors is 2 out of 100,000 people who have high blood pressure. However, some high blood pressure specialists believe that the prevalence of primary hyperaldosteronism is much greater than generally accepted and suggest that

- ✔ As many as one in ten people with high blood pressure have primary hyperaldosteronism (although not necessarily due to a tumor).
- ✔ Primary hyperaldosteronism should be considered in every case of high blood pressure, even when the potassium is normal.
- ✔ Blood tests should determine the ratio of aldosterone and renin levels in the bloodstream.

Whether this high prevalence of primary hyperaldosteronism proves to be a fact isn't clear at this time.

Diagnosing an aldosterone-producing tumor

Aldosterone-producing tumors are usually found in people between the ages of 30 and 50, and they affect women more often than men. People with an aldosterone-producing tumor have the following symptoms:

- ✔ High blood pressure (may be as high as 200/120 mm Hg)
- ✔ Increased potassium in the urine
- ✔ Increased sodium in the blood
- ✔ Increased urination (especially after lying down)
- ✔ Low potassium in the blood, leading to muscle weakness

Because the blood pressure can be so high, people who suffer from an aldosterone-producing tumor may experience a brain attack, damage to the kidneys, or an enlarged heart before the disease is treated (see Part II for more about these consequences of high blood pressure). The low potassium level in the bloodstream can lead to muscle weakness, a reduced secretion of insulin, and diabetes.

Another sign of an aldosterone-producing tumor is a low level of renin versus a significant amount of aldosterone in the bloodstream. Most of the time, elevated aldosterone is secondary to *increased* renin. But with primary hyperaldosteronism, the renin level is low — a sign that an aldosterone-producing tumor (and not renin) is instigating the aldosterone.

(e) (e) (e) hoa .

A kidney with insufficient blood pressure produces renin. As I note in the earlier "Handling blocked kidney arteries" section, the renin causes production of angiotensin II (a strong blood-vessel constriction agent that also triggers the release of aldosterone) from angiotensin I. The elevated blood pressure and increased blood volume result in suppression of renin production. Normally, when a person stands up, renin is released to help increase blood pressure, but because of this tumor, renin doesn't increase with standing.

The following steps explain how a doctor proceeds when he suspects an aldosterone-producing tumor:

1. **High blood pressure is present and a blood test indicates low potassium.**

    (a)

   Sometimes a doctor prescribes a *diuretic* (a drug that promotes the formation of urine by the kidney; see Chapter 13) to lower the blood pressure *before* he considers and tests for an aldosterone-producing tumor. But, because diuretics also push potassium into the urine (reducing the potassium in the bloodstream), they compromise an accurate reading of potassium loss. In this case, the effect of the diuretic must be removed before the blood is tested.

2. **If you have a low blood potassium and an overabundance of potassium in the urine, the doctor orders a blood test for renin.**

   Renin should be especially high if salt and water are withheld.

3. **If the amount of renin in your blood is, in fact, reduced, then your doctor may use that information to screen for an aldosterone-producing tumor by radiologic studies.**

   The aldosterone level should be measured in the early morning because aldosterone tends to fall at night, even from a tumor.

   If the aldosterone level is high, the diagnosis is either an aldosterone-secreting tumor or *bilateral adrenal hyperplasia* — increased aldosterone production in both adrenals as a result of having many nodules. This distinction is important because bilateral adrenal hyperplasia tends to be a milder disease than a tumor, and it doesn't respond well to surgery.

4. **A CT or MRI scan can usually distinguish a solitary adrenal tumor from bilateral hyperplasia.**

   Occasionally, this scan doesn't make the distinction because aldosterone-producing tumors tend to be small and the incidence of *incidentalomas* (innocent growths) on the adrenal gland is high.

5. **If the scan can't distinguish between a tumor and bilateral hyperplasia, the radiologist puts a tube into the adrenal veins on each side of the body and looks for large amounts of aldosterone in the sample.**

   If one side has much aldosterone and the other side doesn't, the diagnosis is an aldosterone-producing tumor, not bilateral hyperplasia.

Lapping up licorice can lower your renin

Believe it or not — eating lots of licorice can raise your blood pressure and lower the amount of renin in your bloodstream. An abundance of licorice can block the enzyme that normally converts cortisol (which maintains blood glucose and helps maintain blood pressure) to cortisone (an anti-inflammatory hormone) in the kidney. Because cortisol has some activity similar to aldosterone in test results and cortisone doesn't, the unusually high concentrations of cortisol *clinically* imitate aldosterone excess. However, a more accurate picture can be drawn from a patient's history of licorice eating and his low aldosterone test results. Don't worry though; the excess usually requires four weeks of eating large quantities (50 to 100 grams) of licorice.

Treating an aldosterone-producing tumor

The treatment of a solitary adrenal tumor that makes too much aldosterone is laparoscopic surgery to remove the tumor. Before surgery, the doctor prescribes *spironolactone,* a drug that reverses the action of aldosterone, for several days to make the patient chemically normal.

After surgery, the aldosterone level falls, the potassium returns to normal, and the blood pressure returns to normal. Sometimes the blood pressure stays up because the patient also has *essential high blood pressure* (high blood pressure for which the cause can't be determined) or because permanent damage has taken place in the blood vessels or the kidneys. This problem occurs most often with individuals who've had high blood pressure for five years or longer.

Usually, doctors don't recommend medical treatment (spironolactone*)* to reverse the action of aldosterone — particularly in men — because the treatment has significant side effects including breast enlargement, reduced interest in sex, and reduced ability to have an erection. Many patients with a single tumor, however, can't undergo surgery for some reason or refuse surgery. In this situation, medical treatment has been successful for five years or more.

Note: If the diagnosis is bilateral adrenal hyperplasia (see Steps 4 and 5 in the previous list), the doctor treats it medically with spironolactone. (Removal of the adrenal glands doesn't generally cure the high blood pressure even though the low potassium improves.)

A new drug, *eplerenone,* is now the drug of choice for bilateral adrenal hyperplasia and *adrenal adenomas* (a tumor in one adrenal gland) because it reverses the low potassium and the high blood pressure without causing the sexual side effects of spironolactone.

Managing Cushing's syndrome

As if the previous two tumors weren't enough trouble from the adrenal gland, the adrenal gland can be the site of still another secondary high blood pressure source, *Cushing's syndrome,* where the adrenal glands make too much cortisol (their main hormone). This syndrome can originate in three different ways:

✔ In about 80 percent of the cases, an excessive production of *adrenocorti-cotrophin* (ACTH, the pituitary hormone that regulates the adrenal gland) caused by a tumor in the pituitary, stimulates both adrenals to make too much cortisol. If a tumor forms in the pituitary gland, it can cause the adrenals to make too much cortisol and other steroids that have plenty of salt-retaining activity. As a result, the blood pressure rises.

✔ In the remaining 20 percent of cases, a tumor grows within one adrenal gland. When the adrenal tumor makes too much cortisol independently of ACTH, the ACTH is suppressed instead of elevated.

✔ Rarely (less than 2 percent), an adrenal-stimulating hormone from some other tumor in the body (particularly a lung cancer) stimulates the adrenals. This condition is *ectopic* (from an abnormal site) ACTH production. The result is Cushing's syndrome, but it tends to be more aggressive, producing low potassium levels. The ectopic source often has some identifying symptom such as cough from a lung cancer.

Diagnosing Cushing's syndrome

Cushing's syndrome is associated with high blood pressure that's difficult to treat. The pressure may be up to 200/120 mm Hg. The syndrome occurs three times more often in women than in men and usually in a person's third or fourth decade. The death rate from untreated Cushing's syndrome is high, approximately 13 percent.

Too much cortisol in the bloodstream has other properties that may result in

✔ Diabetes mellitus (diabetic kidney disease; see the sidebar "The details of diabetic kidney disease" earlier in this chapter for more information)

✔ Easy bruising of the body

✔ Loss of bone, which causes spontaneous fractures

✔ Obesity of the trunk of the body, thin arms and legs

✔ Psychological changes ranging from irritability to severe depression

✔ Purplish stretch marks, especially on the abdomen

In addition to high blood pressure, the high ACTH and the pituitary tumor that it represents can cause still other signs and symptoms such as:

- ✔ Headache caused by the pituitary tumor
- ✔ Pigmentation of the body, particularly any stretch marks caused by the ACTH
- ✔ Loss of menstrual function in women due to the adrenals producing excessive amounts of hormones that have masculinizing properties
- ✔ Hairiness in women due to the same masculinizing hormones

Given all these signs and symptoms, Cushing's syndrome is often considered and relatively easy to prove with chemical tests. The following steps explain how your doctor proceeds when he suspects this condition:

1. **The patient takes 1 milligram of *dexamethasone* (a steroid hormone much like cortisol) at midnight.**

2. **The next morning, the patient has a blood test.**

   If Cushing's syndrome is *not* present, that 1 milligram is enough to shut down ACTH, thereby lowering the cortisol in the bloodstream when tested the following morning.

   However, when a pituitary tumor makes ACTH, or an independent tumor of the adrenal gland makes cortisol, the dexamethasone can't shut down cortisol production; the cortisol is still elevated.

In another confirmatory study, the following steps occur:

1. **A 24-hour urine collection is tested.** High cortisol indicates Cushing's syndrome.

2. **When the screening test is positive, a blood test then measures the amount of ACTH in the bloodstream.**

   If the ACTH is high, then a pituitary tumor is suspected. But if the ACTH is low, then an adrenal tumor is most likely the cause.

3. **Following a positive blood test or a positive urine test, the patient has a CT or MRI test.** If ACTH is high, the doctor orders the test on the pituitary; if ACTH is low, the doctor orders the test on the adrenals. The MRI shows a pituitary tumor, but an abdominal CT may show a tumor in an adrenal gland. If an ectopic source of ACTH is suspected, the CT is directed to look for a tumor in the chest and the abdomen.

Treating Cushing's syndrome

The first step in treating Cushing's syndrome is to control the blood pressure with drugs. The use of drugs is the same as for essential high blood pressure (see Chapter 13). After the blood pressure is under control, the treatment is directed to the source of the excess hormone.

(a) hard.

✔ If the pituitary is responsible through an ACTH-producing tumor, the patient undergoes an operation under anesthesia (don't worry, you won't feel a thing) that involves passing a tube through the nose into the pituitary gland for the removal of the tumor. If this isn't successful or feasible, the patient has X-ray therapy to the pituitary.

✔ Sometimes the pituitary can't be treated (for example, if the patient refuses surgery on the brain). Then both adrenal glands are removed by surgery because the hormones from the adrenals are responsible for most of the signs and symptoms. Afterwards, the patient is treated with steroid replacement.

(a)

A complication of this treatment is the growing tumor in the pituitary and an abundance of ACTH. Over a period of ten years or so, the patient's skin shows significant darkening, a condition known as *Nelson's syndrome.* Then the pituitary tumor must be removed because it is enlarging, losing other pituitary hormones, and causing local symptoms like compression on the optic nerve (the nerve for vision).

✔ If the adrenal gland has a tumor that makes too much cortisol independent of ACTH control, that tumor is removed in much the same way as an aldosterone-producing tumor. (See the "Treating an aldosterone-producing tumor" section earlier in this chapter.)

✔ If ACTH has an ectopic source, then the ACTH is often from a cancer, and chemotherapy may be necessary.

After a patient's pituitary tumor is removed, her cortisol may be abnormally low for as long as six months. She may need support from replacement medication to provide the cortisol, which is essential to life. When her own adrenal gland takes over, the medication can be phased out.

Recognizing a Genetic Disease as the Cause for High Blood Pressure

Congenital adrenal hyperplasia, an inherited disease, is the genetic lack of one or more enzymes that eventually change steroids to cortisol in the adrenal glands. This condition leads to an overproduction of other hormones that have properties similar to aldosterone. When the pituitary gland does not detect sufficient cortisol, it sends out more ACTH to stimulate the adrenals, which then enlarge. The two most common forms of congenital adrenal hyperplasia break down into the following categories:

1. The excessive steroids are

   • Aldosterone-like, producing high blood pressure and low potassium

   • Masculinizing, causing masculine changes in baby girls so that their genital organs are something between male and female

- In milder forms, responsible for the early onset of puberty in boys. This symptomatic increase of male hormone activity (like increased hair and menstrual irregularity) can also occur in young girls.

2. The excessive steroids are aldosterone-like, causing high blood pressure and low potassium, but no sex hormones are made. As a result:

   - Menstruation doesn't take place, so the disease is first detected at puberty in a girl.

   - The lack of male hormones in boys leads to abnormal development of the male sexual organs, so the disease is found earlier than in girls.

Although these conditions are rare, they're easily treated if diagnosed early. Both types of patients take cortisol, which shuts off the excessive ACTH and the production of the abnormal steroids. In the second form of congenital adrenal hyperplasia, the patient also takes sex hormones to replace the absent hormones. Because these diseases are hereditary, they occur in certain families more often than others. (The more common form is more often in Ashkenazi Jews; the less common form is more often in Sephardic Jews but in other families as well.) This predictability alerts doctors to look for the condition whenever a new birth occurs in one of these families.

Checking Out Other Causes of Secondary High Blood Pressure

Several other treatable diseases are associated with high blood pressure. Most of them are reversible, and the high blood pressure responds to the correction of the disease unless it's been present for some time.

Coarctation of the aorta

Coarctation of the aorta is a narrowing of the large artery that leaves the heart. Depending on the severity, the narrowing is usually present at birth though not diagnosed until the teenage years. The narrowing is usually close to the beginning of the aorta but below where the artery branches to the arms. The result is high blood pressure in the arms and lower blood pressure in the legs (which the doctor can observe by simply measuring the blood pressure in the arms and the legs).

The narrowing results in the production of a *murmur,* a humming sound, which can be heard with the doctor's stethoscope in the area of the heart. In addition, the doctor is unable to detect a pulse in the groin. The kidneys respond to the lower blood pressure by putting out more renin (see the earlier section "Handling blocked kidney arteries"); the increase leads to even higher blood pressure above the narrowing but not below it.

Children with this condition can have nosebleeds, dizziness, pounding headaches, and, when they exercise, leg cramps.

During a careful first examination of any baby, the doctor feels for the pulses in the feet and notes whether pulses are present or not. If not, the doctor can order further evaluation with a CT or MRI of the chest.

The treatment consists of surgery to open the narrow area or sometimes *balloon angioplasty,* the same technique used to open the narrow blood vessels of the heart. (See the "Treating blocked kidney arteries" section, earlier in this chapter for more on angioplasty.)

If the coarctation isn't treated, the patient may die before the age of 40 from complications of high blood pressure.

Too much or too little thyroid hormone

Both *hyperthyroidism* (too much thyroid hormone) and *hypothyroidism* (too little thyroid hormone) can be associated with high blood pressure. These conditions may be easy to diagnose if the symptoms are significant, but hypothyroidism is often subtle.

- ✔ If the patient has a rapid pulse, weight loss, and sweating in addition to high blood pressure, then hyperthyroidism must be considered.
- ✔ If the patient has high cholesterol and high blood pressure, the diagnosis of hypothyroidism should certainly be considered.

Thyroid disease is so common, and testing for it is so simple, that everyone over age 35 should have a screening blood test. For more information on your thyroid, see my book *Thyroid For Dummies* (Wiley). Screening consists of a thyroid-stimulating hormone-level blood test.

Ask your doctor to screen you for thyroid disease beginning at age 35 and every five years thereafter.

Hyperthyroidism and hypothyroidism can be treated easily:

- **Hyperthyroidism:** Pills to block thyroid hormone production or a dose of radioactive iodine
- **Hypothyroidism:** Replacement thyroid hormone by mouth

  One pill a day keeps the person entirely normal — at least as far as the thyroid is concerned! That's as good a cure as I know.

In both conditions, the blood pressure returns to normal after treatment.

Acromegaly

Acromegaly is a disease resulting from a slow-growing tumor of the pituitary gland that makes too much growth hormone. The excess growth hormone causes sodium retention, high blood pressure, and many other signs:

- The hands and the feet grow thick.
- The lips, nose, and tongue are thick.
- The skin is coarse and oily.
- The body is weak and sweats excessively.
- If the disease begins before the bones close (a person normally grows until the growing ends of bones are eliminated, referred to as the *bones closing*), the patient is extremely tall, often unable to get through doors without stooping way down.

Untreated, acromegaly can cause diabetes, high blood pressure, and heart disease, all resulting in early death. The following steps explain how a doctor proceeds when she suspects acromegaly:

1. **The patient takes glucose (the type of sugar in the blood), and then has a blood test that checks for growth hormone levels.**

2. **If the test shows elevated growth hormone, the next step is a CT of the brain to look for a pituitary tumor.** Sometimes, the pituitary appears normal and other tumors in the body produce growth hormone. In this case, radiologic studies may find a tumor elsewhere in the body.

Drugs are available to treat acromegaly, but they're not entirely successful and have side effects. Instead, surgery is usually recommended. A brain surgeon goes in through the nose and removes the tumor. If the surgery is successful, the skin shows improvement in a few days. It's most successful when the level of growth hormone isn't very high.

When surgery is ineffective, radiation to the pituitary can cure the disease but may also cause the loss of other pituitary functions (like the production of hormones that control the thyroid gland, the adrenal gland, and the genital organs). The blood pressure falls when the growth hormone level becomes normal.

Sleep apnea

Sleep apnea is a condition in which an individual gasps for breath and snores during sleep following several stops in breathing. It's significant when it happens five or more times in an hour. The results of the restless sleep are extreme fatigue during the day, headaches, and a tendency to fall asleep when he doesn't want to such as when driving a car and at work.

Because the lack of breathing occurs many times, the person has a reduction in blood oxygen and an increase in carbon dioxide. The decrease in oxygen causes constriction of the blood vessels with resultant high blood pressure. These people also tend to have increased heart disease.

Sleep apnea is diagnosed in a sleep laboratory where doctors can observe the person sleeping, snoring, and failing to breathe for many periods of time. After the diagnosis, the person wears a mask that provides positive pressure while he sleeps. This pressure keeps the airway open so he doesn't experience breathing loss, loud snoring, or gasping for air. Sleeping is much more restful, and the person doesn't fall asleep during the day. The high blood pressure usually subsides as well. (Talk about a win-win situation!)

If the condition has gone on for a long time, the high blood pressure may continue, and pills may be required to control it.

Brain tumor

Brain tumors increase pressure within the brain and the blood pressure throughout the body. The blood pressure rise may not be constant and may mimic a pheochromocytoma. (See more on pheochromocytomas in the "Finding an epinephrine-producing tumor" section earlier in this chapter.) If the brain tumor can be managed successfully, the high blood pressure returns to normal. If not, blood pressure pills are required to control it.

Burns

The high stress associated with severe burns causes high blood pressure in about 25 percent of severe burn cases. A bad burn also triggers the release of hormones that cause blood vessel constriction. If the patient survives the burn, the blood pressure returns to normal after about two weeks.

Part II
Considering the Medical Consequences

By Rich Tennant

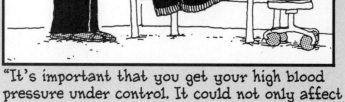

"It's important that you get your high blood pressure under control. It could not only affect your kidney and heart, but also your current brain."

In this part . . .

Three major organs of the body suffer when high blood pressure isn't controlled: the heart, the kidneys, and the brain. In this part, I explain exactly how high blood pressure affects each of these organs and how the sooner any damage is diagnosed, the better the chances are of reversing the damage. I also address ways to deal with organ damage that already exists.

Although I separate these three major organs into separate chapters, uncontrolled high blood pressure doesn't pick and choose. Instead, uncontrolled high blood pressure tends to damage all these organs and within the same time frame.

Chapter 5

Defending Your Heart

*H*eart disease is the leading cause of death throughout the world. It involves the muscles of the heart and the blood vessels that provide nutrition to those muscles. Various forms of heart disease include *angina* (chest pain caused by a decreased blood supply to the heart), heart *failure* (when your heart isn't able to pump enough blood to maintain an adequate flow to and from the body tissues), and heart *attack* (death of heart muscle tissue due to loss of blood supply). High blood pressure plays a major role in the development of heart disease.

High blood pressure without other risk factors such as diabetes, smoking, and lack of exercise is rare. But these risk factors, when mixed in with high blood pressure, can increase the chance of a fatal heart attack as much as 15 to 20 times. In fact, people with untreated high blood pressure may live 10 to 20 years less than people without high blood pressure. When the blood pressure is controlled consistently, however, a person's life span isn't shortened.

It's been said that gambling is a great way of getting nothing for something, and you can gamble away your life if you don't control your blood pressure — this is guaranteed. You must make up your mind to get something for something. Take the trouble to measure your blood pressure properly (see Chapter 2 to find out how) and to follow the recommendations in Part III, and I guarantee that you'll not only live longer but also increase the quality of your life — free of much of the medical misery that people develop as they get older.

This chapter tells you what you need to know about high blood pressure and your heart. It provides a foundation for moving into Part III. If you read this whole chapter, you'll have an excellent understanding of how important blood pressure control is, especially for your heart. The other chapters in this part help you understand how high blood pressure affects your kidneys and your brain.

Even though I discuss the heart, kidneys, and brain in three separate chapters, remember that uncontrolled high blood pressure doesn't just cause the development of heart disease, but also kidney disease and a brain attack as well.

Introducing the Mighty Pump

What a piece of work the heart is! An organ that's mostly muscle, the heart is about the size of a clenched fist and weighs about 10½ ounces. This little muscle is responsible for supplying blood and oxygen (which are usually 15 or more times heavier than the heart itself) to all parts of the body.

Your heart is in your chest cavity behind your breastbone and between your lungs. It's divided into four chambers — the left and right *atria* and the left and right *ventricles.* Here's how the chambers work together:

- ✔ The right atrium receives blood through the *vena cava* (veins) and pushes it into the right ventricle.
- ✔ The right ventricle squeezes down and sends the blood into the pulmonary arteries to the lungs, where the blood picks up oxygen.
- ✔ Pulmonary veins carry the blood back to the left atrium, which sends it down to the left ventricle.
- ✔ The left ventricle squeezes the blood into the *aorta,* a major artery that sends the blood to every cell and organ.
- ✔ Valves that close, blocking backward flow, prevent the blood from going backwards (from the left side of the heart to the lungs, from the right side of the heart to the veins, and from the ventricles to the atria).

This amazing pump pushes 1½ gallons of blood forward every minute. Every hour, it sends 90 gallons around the body, enough to fill a car's 15-gallon gas tank six times. During a fairly restful day, your heart pumps 2,160 gallons of blood. And when you're working or playing energetically, the number gets much higher.

The combination of the heart, the blood vessels that carry the blood, and the blood itself is the *cardiovascular system.*

When the blood pressure rises, the heart must work harder to push the blood through. It wasn't meant to struggle so hard, and eventually it may fail because the heart muscles are just too tired and weak to work properly.

Blocking Blood Flow to the Heart Muscle

Just like any other organ of the body, your heart muscle must receive oxygen, *glucose* (blood sugar), and other nutrients in order to work. These nutrients are the food of the heart muscles. When *arteriosclerosis* (hardening of the arteries) occurs, the bloodstream that carries these nutrients is partially obstructed. The heart muscle then becomes partially starved, which can cause pain. If the obstruction remains about the same, the pain is stable. But a complete obstruction causes a heart attack.

Figure 5-1 shows the location of the major arteries that provide blood supply to the heart muscles.

- The right *coronary* artery supplies blood to the right side of the heart.

- The left *main coronary* artery supplies the left side of the heart. It, in turn, divides into the following:

  - The left *anterior descending* artery that supplies the front of the left side

  - The left *circumflex* artery that curves around to the back

- Both the left and right coronary arteries arise as the left ventricle continues into the aorta.

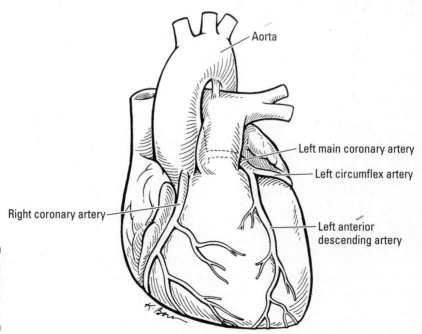

Aorta

Left main coronary artery

Left circumflex artery

Right coronary artery

Left anterior descending artery

Figure 5-1:
Blood
supply to
the heart.

Beware of left ventricular hypertrophy

Under the influence of high blood pressure, heart muscle becomes *hypertrophic,* that is, it begins to thicken just like any muscle that constantly does more work. About 20 percent of people with high blood pressure have *left ventricular hypertrophy,* a severe version of this condition, which can lead to heart attacks or heart failure (both of which I cover later in this chapter). As the muscle gets thicker, it loses its elasticity, leading to reduced blood flow into and out of the heart. The heart begins to enlarge, leading to the need for more blood for the heart tissue, which it can't provide.

Symptoms may include shortness of breath, chest pain, and irregular heartbeats. Your doctor can diagnose left ventricular hypertrophy with an electrocardiogram. Treatment is with blood-pressure-lowering drugs, especially *losartan* (see Chapter 13).

Examining arteriosclerosis

In arteriosclerosis, deposits of cholesterol and formation of a *plaque* (consisting of inflammatory cells and fibrous tissue) cause an artery to narrow, blocking the flow of blood. (See the nearby sidebar "The formation of a plaque" for more information.) When the blood flow is blocked, the heart has to pump harder, leading to *hypertrophy* (thickening of the heart muscles). (See the nearby sidebar "Beware of left ventricular hypertrophy" for details about one kind of hypertrophy.)

High blood pressure can increase the development of fatty deposits in the walls of the arteries, leading to

- **Atherosclerosis:** A form of arteriosclerosis in the medium- to large-size arteries

- **Arteriolosclerosis:** Arteriosclerosis in the small arteries

- **Coronary atherosclerosis:** A form of arteriosclerosis involving the arteries to the muscle of the heart

As the coronary arteries (the ones that feed the heart muscle) become more and more blocked, the heart muscle may become hungry for nutrients or even die, a condition called *coronary artery disease* (also known as *coronary heart disease* and *atherosclerotic heart disease*).

According to the National Institutes of Health, one of every five deaths (460,000 total) in the United States each year is a lethal heart attack as a result of atherosclerosis of the coronary arteries. In addition to these deaths, another 650,000 people have heart attacks but don't die, making a total of about 1.1 million people affected by atherosclerosis each year. About 12.5 million people in the United States have chest pain associated with coronary atherosclerosis, a heart attack, or some other form of coronary atherosclerosis. Due to the greater prevalence of high blood pressure among the African American population, this group has a higher rate of coronary heart disease than any other ethnic group in the United States.

Coronary artery disease has been found in the arteries of people as young as age 20 or younger who die of other causes, and it is extensive in older people who die of other causes. However, not everyone has it. People who don't have risk factors such as uncontrolled high blood pressure, cigarette smoking, diabetes, a sedentary lifestyle, and high cholesterol levels rarely have problems with coronary artery disease. Although a family history of coronary artery disease is another risk factor (and one that you can do nothing about), its effect is minimized when the individual avoids or controls the other risk factors.

Coronary artery disease may cause sudden death as its *first* sign in as many as 25 percent of the patients. Another 20 percent die as a result of a fatal irregularity in their heartbeat before they reach the hospital. The remaining 55 percent may undergo a procedure that tries to open the blocked artery or arteries. (See the "Opting for surgery" section coming up later in this chapter.)

Managing stable heart pain

A large group of patients with coronary artery disease have *angina pectoris* (Latin for *pain in the chest*), a relatively stable form of chest pain that doesn't get worse over time. Commonly known as *angina,* the disease affects 8.9 million people in the United States. It results from blockage of an artery, but it can also occur when the coronary artery squeezes down (after a meal, for example, when blood is diverted to the intestine, thus causing a decrease in blood supply to the heart). Some diseases (such as *hyperthyroidism* — where an overactive thyroid gland increases the demands on the body's metabolism) can cause angina even in the absence of coronary atherosclerosis.

In the following sections, I discuss the symptoms, testing, diagnosis, and treatment of stable heart pain.

Identifying the symptoms

Some of the characteristic symptoms of coronary artery disease include the following:

- ✔ Chest pain begins with activity and is relieved with rest. The person most often feels the pain in the front of the chest on the left side and radiating down the left arm. Even less activity can bring on the pain after a meal or during excitement. Strong emotions can bring on pain even without activity.

- ✔ Symptomatic pain in the chest may be absent. However, according to coronary artery disease patients, symptomatic *discomfort* in the chest area can include burning, squeezing, pressing, aching, or indigestion.

✔ The area of discomfort is most often behind the middle of the chest, and it tends to be in the same area for an individual each time he has it. Other places may include the right side of the chest, the left shoulder, and sometimes the right shoulder. It can also be in the jaw. The discomfort often radiates from one of those sites back to the chest.

✔ Discomfort may last no longer than a few minutes, especially if the patient rests as soon as it starts. It doesn't last longer than 30 minutes.

✔ *Nitroglycerin* often reduces or stops the pain, and this same response helps to make the diagnosis.

The formation of plaque

When high blood pressure, smoking, diabetes, or increased levels of cholesterol (especially low-density lipoprotein [LDL] cholesterol) damage the inner lining of the arteries, a plaque (obstruction) begins to form. The following figure shows the parts of a normal artery before and after plaque develops.

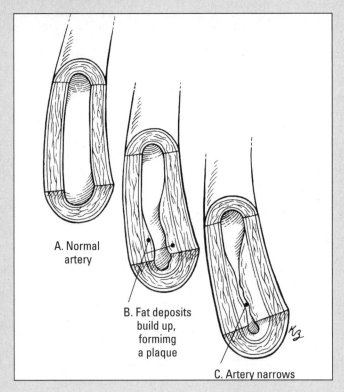

A. Normal artery

B. Fat deposits build up, formimg a plaque

C. Artery narrows

After damage occurs, the following steps take place:

1. Fat begins to accumulate within the *intima,* the innermost part of the artery wall.

2. The chemicals that normally prevent changes to the fat can't reach it — the fat begins to change to a more damaging form.

3. White blood cells enter the intima, transform into *macrophages* (large cells), and begin gobbling up the changed fat, turning the cells into *foam cells.*

   Note: Macrophages normally remove waste products, harmful microorganisms, and foreign material from the bloodstream.

4. Calcium also deposits in the walls of plaque. It's responsible for the calcification in arteries that is visible in X-rays.

5. This accumulation of foam cells and calcium is now plaque. It grows and begins to stick out into the *lumen* (the hollow part) of the artery.

6. Blood flow to the heart muscle is reduced when 80 percent of the lumen is blocked.

7. Blood platelets can accumulate to form clots on the irregular surface of plaque. The clot can stay at that position (reducing the opening of the lumen even more) or break off and lodge in a smaller artery (completely closing off blood flow beyond it).

Testing and making a diagnosis

The doctor may use certain blood tests to characterize the type and extent of the heart disease. These include the following:

- ✓ **Cardiac enzymes:** Blood chemicals that are in higher amounts when the heart damage is acute

- ✓ **C-reactive protein:** A chemical in the blood that indicates you're responding to injury or infection

  High levels indicate an increased risk of a heart attack or brain attack.

- ✓ **Fibrinogen:** A protein that promotes blood clots and is present in higher amounts in higher risk patients

- ✓ **Homocysteine:** A chemical that indicates increased danger of brain attack, heart attack, or blockage of blood vessels to the legs

- ✓ **Low-density cholesterol:** A form of fat in the blood that increases atherosclerosis

The blood levels of these chemicals and the patient's description of symptoms usually lead the doctor to diagnose angina. But the classic diagnostic tool for this condition is a stress test. The patient walks on a treadmill or bikes on a stable bike up to 12 minutes at increasing speeds and increasing slopes while a continuous *electrocardiogram* (EKG — a recording of the electrical impulses in the heart) is performed.

This test is accurate only if the patient achieves a certain level of activity and heart rate and sustains the activity long enough. The doctor looks for specific changes on the graph paper especially if chest pain occurs during the EKG.

When a stress test indicates angina pectoris, other tests that require an intravenous line or even less invasive measures can further characterize the severity of the coronary artery disease. These include the following:

- **Coronary angiogram:** This test is the gold standard for the diagnosis of angina pectoris, and it's ordered when the preceding tests indicate an abnormality. To find the areas of narrowing, the doctor places a catheter in the individual coronary arteries and injects a dye that's visible on an X-ray. Coronary angiography is only for patients who exhibit the following:

  - Stable or unstable angina is present, and medical treatment with pills is unsuccessful.

  - Symptoms don't point to a diagnosis of coronary artery disease.

  - Coronary artery surgery has been performed, but symptoms return.

  - Heart has severe abnormal rhythm disturbances that may be caused by coronary artery disease.

- **Echocardiography:** Using sound to bounce off the walls of the heart, this test shows areas that don't contract with the rest of the heart muscle. A device that sends a sound wave to the heart muscle is held over your heart, producing a picture of the moving heart muscle. This is truly *noninvasive* to your body.

- **Myocardial perfusion scan:** This test shows where the myocardium (heart muscle) is and isn't receiving normal blood flow. After a radioactive tracer is injected through an IV, and an instrument similar to a Geiger counter for detecting radioactivity locates the tracer in the heart. When no radioactivity is observed, no *perfusion* (blood delivery) is occurring.

- **Radionuclide angiography:** This test measures the *ejection fraction* (the amount of blood that's pushed out of the heart with each beat divided by the amount of blood within the left ventricle when it's completely full) and the motion of the heart wall to identify which areas may have lost their blood supply and are probably dead tissue.

The ejection fraction should rise with exercise, but when coronary artery disease is present, it may fall. (See the later sidebar "Ejection fraction, what's your function?" for more information.) A radioactive substance that attaches to red blood cells is injected into your blood through an IV. The radioactivity is counted as it goes through your heart.

After a coronary angiogram clearly points to obstructive coronary artery disease, the doctor determines a treatment plan.

Treating with medication

Three major forms of treatment are available for coronary artery obstruction, and each has its advantages and disadvantages. One treatment option for patients with stable, uncomplicated angina pectoris is medication. This option is usually best for patients who aren't interested in exertion. However, if the patient wants to perform energetic activities or has unstable angina, then two surgical procedures — *percutaneous transluminal coronary angioplasty* (PTCA) or *coronary artery bypass graft* (CABG) — are the treatments of choice. (I discuss them in the following section.)

Before prescribing drugs, the doctor wants to eliminate contributing factors. (See "Avoiding the Risk Factors" later in this chapter.) If blood pressure is high, it must be brought under control. If the patient smokes, he must stop. Diabetes needs to be controlled, and elevated cholesterol need to be treated.

Strenuous activity may provoke pain, which may have to be eliminated as well. A number of drugs have successfully reduced pain and increased the time that such patients can exercise without it recurring. For example:

- **Beta blockers,** a class of drugs in pill form that include *propranolol, metoprolol,* and *atenolol,* decrease the heart's oxygen requirements, thereby decreasing pain. **Note:** Beta blockers actually prolong the life of angina sufferers.

- **Calcium channel-blocking agents,** another class of drugs such as *verapamil* and *diltiazem,* reduce the heart's oxygen needs by reducing blood pressure and heart rate. They are in pill form.

- **Drugs that dilate the blood vessels or prevent the blood's platelets from forming a clot** (such as aspirin) can reduce pain and prevent further clotting. These are available in pill form.

- **Long-acting nitrates** such as *isosorbide dinitrate* and *isosorbide mononitrate* decrease the frequency of pain attacks. In addition to pills, they're available as a patch that's worn during the day; the medication is absorbed through the skin.

- **Nitroglycerin** has been successful for years. It opens up the arteries directly and lowers the blood pressure so the heart doesn't have to work as hard. Nitroglycerin is placed under the tongue at the first sign of pain and usually works in minutes.

Opting for surgery

As I mention earlier in this section, two surgical procedures that treat coronary artery obstruction include PTCA and CABG.

Studies of patients who were randomly given PTCA or CABG show similar results. For a single blocked blood vessel, the two operations have equal rates of success. **Note:** This similarity is also true for multiple vessels as long as the patient isn't diabetic and the obstructed blood vessels can be entered. In the latter case, however, bypass surgery is the treatment of choice.

For PTCA you are awake. Your groin area is cleaned and numbed. A tiny incision allows the cardiologist to find an artery so he can place a guide wire and a tube up to the blockage in the coronary artery. The doctor observes the blocked artery by injecting dye through the tube and taking an X-ray. He then inflates a balloon at that end of the tube to widen the area of blockage and stretch it out. This step may be repeated, and the tube and balloon are then removed. After the blockage is open, the doctor may also place a *stent* (an open tubular structure made of metal) at that location to act like a scaffold and keep the artery open. By using certain drugs on the stent, the blockage remains open much longer. You may be in the hospital a day and return to work the next week. Some recent research suggests that drug-coated stents may cause death earlier than non-drug-coated stents.

For CABG, you're under general anesthesia and a large incision is made to open the chest. The flow of blood is diverted from the heart to a heart-lung machine, which provides blood to the rest of the body while the heart is still. The surgeon attaches a healthy blood vessel (from the leg or the inside of the chest) onto both sides of the blocked artery. The blood then flows freely through that blood vessel. The surgery takes up to six hours because two to four arteries are repaired. You're usually in the intensive care unit for a couple of days, out of the hospital by a week after surgery, and back to work in 6 to 12 weeks.

PTCA has a number of advantages over CAGB:

- ✔ PTCA is a simpler surgery and doesn't require anesthesia.
- ✔ The chest isn't opened up.
- ✔ The heart isn't bypassed during surgery.
- ✔ Convalescence is relatively short, and the usual discharge occurs after 24 hours.

However, in general, CAGB lasts longer and provides a more complete reopening of blood flow. In addition, two newer procedures make your stay in the hospital much shorter following CAGB:

✔ Using *beating-heart* surgery, the surgeon stills only the area of the heart that he's operating on. This improvement results in much less overall trauma, which shortens the hospital stay.

✔ The surgeon uses much smaller incisions in the chest, making this surgery minimally invasive, especially when only one artery needs opening.

Disadvantages and complications accompany each procedure:

✔ PTCA can't be performed when an artery is completely closed. Also, PTCA isn't effective when many separate lesions are present. This problem may be the reason PTCA isn't the treatment of choice for diabetics with coronary artery disease, where multiple arteries are affected. These patients do much better with CABG.

✔ CABG can have complications (an acute heart attack, a stroke, an infection in the body's surgical site, and even death on the operating table), especially in patients more than 70 years old and patients with other diseases such as kidney disease and diabetes (check out the later section "Controlling diabetes"). In these patients, CABG is only performed when symptoms are most severe (for example, unremitting chest pain).

Treating a heart attack

A *myocardial infarction* (MI) is a heart attack where heart muscle tissue dies because it lacks a supply of blood. It can cause immediate death in 25 percent of the people who have one, and another 20 percent never reach the hospital alive. For those who do make it to the hospital, however, excellent treatment is available.

The symptoms that suggest that an individual is having a heart attack include the following:

✔ Development of severe pain in the front of the chest that lasts for more than 30 minutes with radiation down the left arm

✔ Unexplained shock or a severe fall in blood pressure, sometimes accompanied by vomiting and even unconsciousness

✔ A feeling of impending doom with sweating and a rapid heartbeat

Call 911 for an ambulance ride to the nearest hospital, and call your doctor for follow-up.

The doctor will ask whether you've had a recent change in your pattern of chest pain and whether you're experiencing sweating, dizziness, nausea, and weakness.

In addition:

- ✔ Your blood pressure may be low.
- ✔ You may appear pale.
- ✔ Your heart rhythm may be irregular.
- ✔ Your heart may reveal soft sounds that mean the muscle isn't functioning properly.

  On examination, your chest may have *rales,* the sound of fluid in the lungs as a result of some heart failure (see the next section for more information).

The doctor does lab studies, which may show the following:

- ✔ **Elevations of heart enzymes,** chemicals (usually found only in the heart) that leak into the blood when the heart muscle is damaged.
- ✔ **Electrocardiographic changes** that suggest a heart attack.
- ✔ **Changes in the movement of the heart wall;** the wall doesn't move at all, or it may flop outward when it should be moving in to squeeze out blood.

See the earlier section "Testing and making a diagnosis" for more on each of these studies.

One of the biggest advances in the treatment of heart attacks is the availability of *thrombolytic therapy,* intravascular drugs that dissolve the clot that's obstructing the coronary artery, thereby allowing blood to flow back into the obstructed area. This treatment decreases the size of the damage and often saves the patient. *Note:* A possible side effect of thrombolytic therapy is the danger of bleeding in undesired areas such as the brain — especially when the blood pressure isn't controlled.

Doctors can use several different agents for thrombolytic therapy, and the choice depends on your doctor's experience with each of them. But the success of this treatment depends on how quickly the patient gets to the doctor after the onset — the earlier, the better. The reopening may be as much as 80 percent, and it accompanies an end to the pain and an improved EKG reading.

After the initial therapy, the heart attack patient remains in the coronary care unit for a couple of days and gradually returns to normal activity.

If the blood vessel closes again (this happens in 10 percent of cases), the patient must have PTCA or CABG to reopen the artery permanently. (I describe these two procedures in the previous section.) Sometimes the doctor chooses immediate PTCA over thrombolytic therapy, especially in the severely sick patient with a heart attack and shock.

Studies have shown that several drugs can significantly reduce the chance of a future heart attack when they're prescribed early. For example:

- ✔ Aspirin to prevent more clots
- ✔ Beta blockers to extend the life of the patient
- ✔ Nitroglycerine as the treatment of choice when pain occurs

Developing Heart Failure

Heart failure is clearly more prevalent today compared to 25 years ago. The reason for the increase isn't clear, but uncontrolled high blood pressure is certainly one contributing factor.

When high blood pressure is present, your heart is forced to pump against more resistance. To sustain its output, the heart gets bigger and thicker, just like the muscles of a weight lifter. But heart muscle can only thicken so much. After a while, it's too large to pump effectively, and heart failure begins.

If you suffer from heart failure, you may experience pain in the front of the chest, the jaw, the left arm, or the shoulder. I describe this pain (angina) earlier in this chapter in the "Managing stable heart pain" section. This pain comes from the high oxygen requirement of the thick heart muscle plus the decreased blood supply coming through the arteries that supply the heart.

Your doctor can tell that your heart is developing problems because he hears the changes in your heart sounds through his stethoscope. Also, with his hand on the front of your chest, he can feel your heart thumping against the chest wall. As your heart fails, that thumping moves away from the center of your chest, indicating that your heart is getting larger.

In this section, I discuss the signs and symptoms of heart failure as well as the many options for its treatment after your doctor has made a definite diagnosis.

Noticing the telltale signs

The most common symptom of heart failure is *dyspnea* (difficulty breathing). At first, breathing is only difficult during exercise. As heart failure increases, however, the individual has difficulty breathing when she's resting, too. ***Note:*** People without heart failure may get short of breath with exercise, too, but only *after* exercising at least a few minutes or so. People whose hearts are failing have difficulty breathing *at the onset* of exercising.

Dyspnea develops when the blood vessels of the failing heart become congested with blood — sometimes even leaking into the lung tissue. The lungs, ordinarily light and filled with air, become much heavier. The diaphragm and other muscles of respiration have a much harder time pushing air out and pulling it in. As they become fatigued, the person experiences shortness of breath.

The patient is unable to lie down flat without raising his head because more blood pools in the lungs, making breathing even more difficult. As a result, the patient may need to sleep on several pillows. If his head falls off the pillows, he may have *orthopnea,* a coughing spell that improves when the patient sits up or raises his head.

Sometimes a severe coughing spell and shortness of breath that can't be relieved just by sitting up or raising the head can awaken the patient. This can be a terrifying experience because the patient can't catch his breath. This *paroxysmal nocturnal dyspnea* is associated with an abundance of fluid in the lung tissue.

Symptoms as severe as paroxysmal nocturnal dyspnea require a call to 911 and emergency room treatment.

Other less specific signs and symptoms of heart failure include:

- ✔ Fatigue and weakness
- ✔ Confused mental state due to poor blood flow to the brain

Severe shortness of breath, mental confusion, severe fatigue, or the new onset of chest pain requires a visit to your doctor.

Understanding what the doctor looks for

The following list presents some of the signs and symptoms that the doctor looks for when she suspects that heart failure is present. But you, too, can recognize many of these if you or a loved one has heart failure:

- ✔ **Swollen legs:** The legs swell because of *edema* (water in the tissues; you can see a dent when the finger pushes into the skin).

- ✔ **Large liver:** A tender, large liver fills with fluid.

- ✔ **Jaundice:** Yellow eyes and yellow skin characterize this condition. The yellowing is a result of severe liver damage due to fluid in the liver.

- ✔ **Off-beat heart sounds:** Your doctor hears abnormal heart sounds with her stethoscope.

- ✔ **Rales:** These crackling sounds in the lungs indicate the presence of fluid in the lung tissue.

- ✔ **Swollen abdomen:** The abdomen swells because of fluid in the abdominal cavity.

- ✔ **Decreased urine flow:** Due to diminished blood flow to the kidneys, the body's normal production of urine decreases.

- ✔ **Cold and pale limbs:** Arms and legs are cold and pale because of poor blood flow.

As you can tell, this is a description of a very sick individual. Patients may have one or more of these symptoms. You don't want this to be what you see in the mirror some day! Start following the recommendations in Part III right away to lower your blood pressure and decrease your chances of developing heart failure.

Ejection fraction, what's your function?

Assessing the *ejection fraction* is one of the best ways to measure your heart function. The ejection fraction is the resulting ratio when the *stroke volume* (amount of blood that's pushed out of the heart with each beat) is divided by the *end diastolic volume* (amount of blood within the large chamber of the heart, the left ventricle, when it's completely full). If the ejection fraction is low (for example less than 50 percent), a significant fraction of the blood in the left ventricle is left inside the heart with each beat, suggesting an inefficient (failing) heart. These volumes can be determined by an ultrasound study that uses the different echo properties of blood and heart tissue to produce a picture of the heart at rest *(end diastolic volume)* or when pumping *(end systolic volume)*. The amount of blood at rest minus the amount after pumping, divided by the amount at rest, gives the ejection fraction. Alternately, an X-ray study can provide the same information.

Measurements while the patient is exercising may be even more helpful because this is the time when the heart is being maximally stressed. Although unstressed values may be normal, the patient may show evidence of significant heart failure when the heart is stressed.

A chest X-ray and an EKG can help your doctor see the severity of the heart failure. These standard tests are ordered for most types of heart disease including heart failure.

- **Chest X-ray:** This test indicates the size of the heart and the presence and extent of fluid in the lungs. Often the veins in the chest are visible in the X-ray because the backed-up blood enlarges these veins.

- **Electrocardiogram:** This test may indicate an enlarged heart, but often other testing shows more.

Treating heart failure

After heart failure is diagnosed, your doctor gives you the information and the drugs you need to manage the condition. This complicated process can't be discussed in detail here. See *Heart Disease For Dummies* by James M. Rippe, MD (Wiley), for more information on this treatment. However, like all illness, successful treatment depends on your willingness to follow the doctor's recommendations. Some of your doctor's instructions and treatments may include the following:

- Significant reduction in salt intake, not just to lower blood pressure but even more importantly to prevent water retention associated with increased salt (see Chapter 10 for more information on limiting your salt intake)

- Use of certain medications including

  - A drug from the category of *ACE inhibitors* (see Chapter 13) to help lower blood pressure and reduce salt and water retention early in the development of heart failure

  - *Diuretics* to eliminate salt and water through the kidneys

  - *Vasodilators* to open the arteries

  - *Digitalis,* a drug that increases the heart muscle's ability to contract

- Restriction of activity to give the heart a rest

- Weight loss to reduce the work of the heart (I discuss weight loss in Chapter 9)

- Reduction of fluid intake to no more than 48 ounces daily.

Avoiding the Risk Factors

Uncontrolled high blood pressure makes both heart failure and heart attacks much more difficult to manage, so controlling the high blood pressure is an early step toward managing these complications.

Some risk factors that contribute to high blood pressure can't be avoided (like family history of early heart disease). But doing everything possible to avoid or eliminate other risk factors helps to prevent heart failure and heart attacks — two complications of high blood pressure — and minimize their impact if they do occur. In the following sections, I point out how prevalent these risk factors remain, how much of a role they continue to play in the occurrence of heart failure and heart attacks, and their prognoses when they do occur.

Curbing high cholesterol

Half of the United States adult population has abnormally high cholesterol levels. These statistics are similar for the United Kingdom, Australia, and New Zealand. For a breakdown of the various ethnic populations, the rates are

- **Caucasian:** 52 percent of men and 49 percent of women
- **African American:** 45 percent of men and 46 percent of women
- **Hispanic:** 53 percent of men and 48 percent of women
- **Native American:** 38 percent of men and 37 percent of women

Given these numbers, it's astonishing that doctors don't see far more patients with complications, especially heart attacks in association with high blood pressure.

High cholesterol is treatable. The dietary changes I recommend in Chapter 9 along with the exercise recommendations of Chapter 12 can take care of most cases. In addition, cholesterol that doesn't respond to diet and exercise is easily managed by *statins,* a powerful group of cholesterol-lowering drugs.

Find out the level of your cholesterol and bring it down. The lower your cholesterol, the better.

Cutting tobacco use

In many ways, tobacco use is a greater problem than high cholesterol. The most important reason is that you're addicted to cigarettes, but you're not addicted to fat. Breaking the smoking habit is difficult but definitely worth the effort.

About a quarter of the United States population is addicted to cigarette smoking. The ethnic breakdown is

- ✔ **Caucasian:** 26 percent of men and 24 percent of women
- ✔ **African American:** 29 percent of men and 21 percent of women
- ✔ **Hispanic:** 25 percent of men and 13 percent of women
- ✔ **Native American:** 42 percent of men and 38 percent of women

Just how many men and women continue to commit slow suicide is astonishing. Even more astonishing is the rate of cigarette smoking among young people who are very much aware of the statistics that relate cigarettes not only to heart disease, but also to emphysema, lung cancer, and many other cancers.

In Chapter 11, I provide everything researchers know about how to stop smoking — one of the most difficult tasks you may ever face. In terms of the benefits to your health, though, nothing you do can be of greater value.

Controlling diabetes

Today more than 21 million Americans have diabetes. That's 5 million (more than 30 percent) more than in 2002, when I wrote the first edition of this book! Heart attacks remain the most frequent cause of death among diabetics, and they're responsible for two-thirds of all deaths among diabetics. They also tend to be more complicated than a heart attack in a nondiabetic. For example, the extensive nature of the *atherosclerotic plaque* (areas of obstruction in blood vessels) in diabetics results in a poor response to PTCA surgery and the need for CABG (a more invasive surgery) when angina or a heart attack occurs. (See the earlier section "Opting for surgery" for more details about PTCA and CABG.)

The prognosis is less pessimistic when the diabetes is under control. This means keeping the blood glucose as close to the normal range as possible (between 80 and 120 milligrams of glucose per deciliter of blood [mg/dL]) and keeping the *hemoglobin A1c* (a test for long-term diabetic control) less than 7 percent of the total hemoglobin.

Diabetes is the diagnosis when the blood glucose is 126 mg/dL on two or more occasions in the fasting state or 200 mg/dL in a random blood glucose check on two or more occasions. However, the patient already has *impaired* fasting glucose (impaired glucose tolerance) at 100 to 126 in the fasting state or 140 to 200 at random. The increased risk of heart disease associated with the blood glucose is present at these lower levels of blood glucose as well. The number of people with these conditions isn't small either. The United States statistics for just impaired fasting glucose are as follows:

- ✔ **Caucasian:** 9 percent of men and 5 percent of women
- ✔ **African American:** 3 percent of men and 5 percent of women
- ✔ **Hispanic:** 12 percent of men and 7 percent of women

The solution is to keep your weight down, get plenty of exercise, avoid fats, and keep your blood glucose under 100 fasting or 140 random. These steps keep your heart risk at a minimum. See my book *Diabetes For Dummies,* 2nd Edition (Wiley) for full details on controlling diabetes.

Stepping up physical activity

Lack of physical activity is clearly a risk factor for heart disease, as much as tobacco smoking. Because many people do work that requires little physical activity, they need to exercise during their leisure time. However, this proactive approach isn't happening. The following percentages show the populations that don't exercise regularly:

- ✔ **Caucasian:** 33 percent of men and 39 percent of women
- ✔ **African American:** 46 percent of men and 57 percent of women
- ✔ **Hispanic:** 50 percent of men and 57 percent of women

Anyone who says that Americans are on the move hasn't looked at these numbers! Chapter 12 tells you how to get going and keep going. The farther you walk, the longer you live. It's as simple as that.

Chapter 6

Shielding Your Kidneys

· ·

· ·

*A*lthough I discuss how high blood pressure affects the heart, kidneys, and brain in three separate chapters, this doesn't mean that individuals with high blood pressure develop only one of the diseases — heart disease *or* kidney disease *or* a brain attack. Uncontrolled high blood pressure triggers their developments all at the same time, so all these complications may progress together. Other factors may prevent a heart attack or brain attack (such as taking aspirin), allowing kidney disease to dominate the picture, or a patient may have only two complications at the same time for some other reason. Still, you can prevent all these complications if you control your blood pressure.

This chapter discusses the kidney and how high blood pressure damages it. I cover how the damage occurs, how it proceeds, and how it leads to end-stage renal disease if unchecked. If you read this whole chapter, I expect that you'll have the same great appreciation for your kidneys that I have for mine. You may even raise a glass of water and toast them!

Don't accept a diagnosis of high blood pressure until you've had multiple high readings, and even then, measure your blood pressure at home with a reliable monitor (see Chapter 2) both to confirm the diagnosis and to follow your body's response to treatment. After high blood pressure is verified, it's usually persistent. However, high blood pressure may improve, especially when a person makes lifestyle changes, even though some damage to the kidneys is permanent.

Examining the Role of Your Kidneys

Your body has two kidneys, each weighing about 6 ounces (or less than ½ of 1 percent of the body's total weight). Each kidney is about 4 inches high, 2 inches wide, and 1 inch thick. Figure 6-1 shows their position in your abdomen.

Blood enters the kidneys through the large *renal arteries.* The *renal cortex* is the kidney's outer shell that contains blood vessels and urine tubes. The *renal pyramids,* the innermost tissue of the kidneys, contain the urine tubes and the specialized tissue that permits fine-tuning of the various substances that leave the kidneys in the urine. Figure 6-2 shows an inside view of the kidney's major parts.

In the following sections, I describe the kidneys' various functions including filtering, renin production, and hormone production.

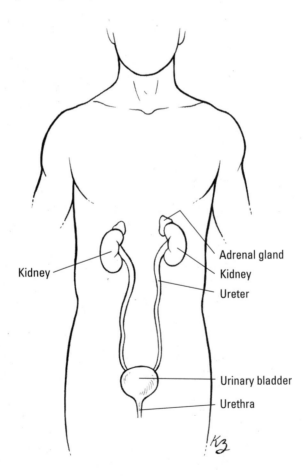

Adrenal gland

Kidney

Kidney

Ureter

Urinary bladder

Urethra

Figure 6-1:
The position
of the
kidneys.

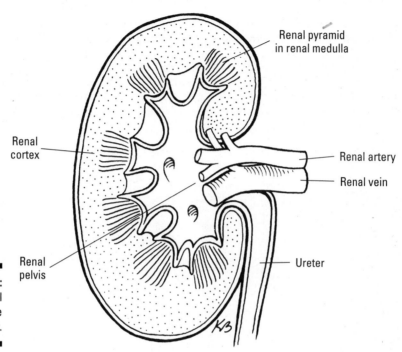

Renal pyramid
in renal medulla

Renal
cortex

Renal artery

Renal vein

Renal
pelvis

Ureter

Figure 6-2:
The internal
parts of the
kidney.

Focusing on the filtering function

Your kidneys are truly amazing. The digestive tract only takes out the waste
that goes through the digestive tract, but the kidneys filter the blood,
which acts much like a cargo carrier as it picks up waste from all the cells
in your body. The blood carries the waste to your body's waste-disposal
headquarters — the kidneys.

Your kidneys filter an enormous amount of blood every minute, about 1½
quarts. During this process, the kidneys filter out blood cells (such as your
red and white blood cells) and large chemical compounds for recycling. But
everything else, including the toxins (normal waste products), makes the
trip. In the next step:

- ✔ A little water carries the toxins to the bladder as urine, which then
  passes out of the body through the urethra.

- ✔ The kidneys reabsorb the recyclable materials — 99 percent of the
  desired water, sodium, and other key body elements — back into
  the body.

Note: The blood that enters the kidneys in the renal (kidney) arteries makes its way through smaller and smaller arteries that eventually branch into capillaries (the human body's smallest blood vessels). But just before passing into a capillary, blood goes through the *afferent arteriole,* the tiny artery that brings blood to the *nephron* (the kidney's filtering device; see Figure 6-3). Each kidney contains 1 million nephrons. After filtering takes place, the liquid part of the blood (with all its dissolved elements — sodium, potassium, uric acid, and many others) passes through these capillaries into the *efferent arteriole.*

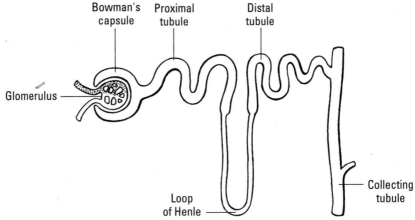

Figure 6-3:
The
nephron: A
unique filter.

The capillary network within the nephron is the *glomerulus.* The *Bowman's capsule,* a bulb that surrounds the glomerulus, receives all the filtered water and begins returning most of it to the bloodstream. At the same time, this bulb releases all the unnecessary substances as urine into the *collecting tubule,* which then empties the urine into the *renal pelvis.* In the final step, the urine travels through the *ureter* to the bladder (refer to Figure 6-2 to see the renal pelvis and the ureter). Whew!

Because this entire process requires pressure to force the liquid part of the blood, the kidney has a *renin-angiotensin-aldosterone system,* a built-in mechanism (see Chapter 4) that maintains the necessary level of blood pressure. But too much pressure for too much time causes damage. And if the damage proceeds, the result is end-stage renal disease where the kidneys can't filter the blood or eliminate toxins without the help of dialysis or transplantation. (For more on dialysis and kidney transplants, see the "Coping with End-Stage Renal Disease" section later in this chapter.)

Understanding other kidney functions

In addition to filtering out and passing off your body's waste, your kidneys affect your blood pressure in other ways, too. This section covers two critical problems: your kidneys' overproduction of *renin* (an enzyme) and complications of hormone imbalances.

Renin production

The *juxtaglomerular cells* are adjacent to the afferent arterioles — the small blood vessels that carry blood to the kidney's filtering site. But when the arterioles detect that the blood pressure is insufficient for filtration to take place, the juxtaglomerular cells go into action and release renin, which eventually leads to the production of angiotensin II (for more on this process, see Chapter 4). This development has two effects:

- ✔ **Blood vessel constriction:** The blood pressure immediately rises.

- ✔ **Aldosterone secretion:** Blood pressure rises even higher because this secretion causes salt and water retention.

Is the kidney the source of most high blood pressure?

Studies show that high blood pressure damages the kidneys, but what causes the onset of essential (unknown cause) high blood pressure?

Many scientists insist that the kidneys are the source of essential high blood pressure, citing a study in *Circulation Research* (June 1975) involving an experiment on rats with hereditary high blood pressure. The results show:

- ✔ If a rat from a strain that's known to have normal blood pressure throughout life has its kidneys removed and receives a normal kidney from a strain that's known to develop high blood pressure later in life, the rat develops high blood pressure.

- ✔ When a rat that's prone to high blood pressure in the future has its kidneys removed and receives a normal kidney from a normal rat, high blood pressure doesn't develop.

Therefore, the study concludes, the glitch must be somewhere in the kidneys of the high blood pressure strain; even when a kidney from the strain of rats with high blood pressure has normal appearance and hasn't been subjected to high blood pressure as yet, it brings on high blood pressure.

The rat study's main conclusion? Rats with hereditary high blood pressure lose the ability to excrete salt from their body at a young age. This salt retention leads to water retention and a subsequent rise in blood pressure.

After the juxtaglomerular cells perceive a satisfactory blood pressure, they stop making renin.

Hormone production

Specialized cells within the kidneys produce *erythropoietin,* a hormone that stimulates the bone marrow to make more red blood cells. Whenever blood is lost or a trip to high altitude demands more oxygen, the need for red blood cells is greater, so the kidneys produce erythropoietin. However, if kidney damage occurs, the cells that make erythropoietin decline, and *anemia* (a fall in the oxygen-carrying red blood cells) develops.

Another important function of the kidneys is the production of *1,25 dihydroxy vitamin D,* a hormone that stimulates the uptake of calcium in the intestine. This hormone is actually the active end-product of vitamin D3 as a result of these steps:

1. The process begins in the skin, where vitamin D is turned into vitamin D3 by the ultraviolet rays of the sun.

2. This substance then circulates to the liver, where it's converted to the next stage of active vitamin D3 production, 25 hydroxy vitamin D.

3. Finally, it reaches the kidneys, where the most active form is produced.

When kidney function declines, highly active vitamin D3 declines. As a result, calcium isn't taken up in sufficient quantities, causing *osteomalacia,* the formation of poorly calcified, weak bones.

Damaging the Kidney

Using renin, aldosterone, heart muscles, and many other tools in the body, the kidneys attempt to regulate the blood pressure at the glomerulus (see the earlier section "Focusing on the filtering function" for more on this capillary network). The pressure needs to be high enough to push out the water and dissolved substances, but not so high that it damages the glomerular cells.

When this regulation fails, kidney damage begins. As kidney tissue is lost, each remaining glomerulus must filter more. As a result, pressure at the glomerulus rises and does even more damage. This increased pressure maintains short-term kidney function but creates more long-term damage.

Plenty of experimental evidence suggests that higher pressure in the glomerulus damages the kidney:

- ✔ If 90 percent of an animal's kidney is removed, the increased pressure damages the remaining glomeruli.

- ✔ When animals are fed a protein-restricted diet, which lowers glomerular blood pressure, the damage slows.

- ✔ Drugs that lower glomerular pressure in humans, even without lowering pressure in the arm, slow the onset of damage.

- ✔ Drugs that lower arm pressure in animals but don't lower the glomerular pressure don't protect the kidneys.

Just exactly *how* increased blood pressure in the glomeruli leads to kidney damage is unclear at this point. Current research suggests that the pressure causes production of certain chemicals that stimulate cell growth in the glomerulus and injure normal cells. The *endothelial cells* (cells that line the inside of blood vessels) may be the source because they make nitric oxide (an important substance that widens blood vessels) and chemicals that may damage the blood vessels. As more cells grow in the tiny space of the glomerulus, the surface area decreases, thereby limiting the amount of blood that can be filtered.

If kidney damage is suspected, your doctor will do blood tests for the levels of *urea nitrogen* (BUN) and *creatinine* as well as urine tests to measure the amount of function that remains in your kidneys. ***Note:*** One very important test is measurement of *albumin* (protein) in the urine. More than 300 milligrams daily suggests a more rapid loss of kidney function. In addition, the doctor will do visual studies of the kidneys to further define the amount of kidney loss and to help diagnose the reason for the kidney failure. These studies include

- ✔ Ultrasound of the kidneys, which shows their size and shape

- ✔ Kidney biopsy, which identifies the exact disease that is causing the damage

- ✔ Computerized tomography, which gives a more detailed picture of the kidneys than a regular X-ray

- ✔ Magnetic Resonance Imaging, which can show the kidneys in cross-section

- ✔ Renal arteriogram, which shows the appearance of the kidney arteries and any obstruction within them

- ✔ An isotopic scan of the kidneys, which provides info on blood flow to the kidneys and the kidney function

Life before and after miracle drugs

Before medications for high blood pressure control were available, researchers studied and followed a great number of people with uncontrolled high blood pressure. After 15 to 25 years of no control, about 40 percent of the patients had abnormally high levels of protein (an indication of kidney damage) in their urine. They lived about 5 years longer. Patients that had an elevation in blood urea nitrogen (evidence of kidney function loss) lived about another year.

A typical study is in the *Journal of Chronic Diseases* (January 1955), where 500 patients were followed for an average of 20 years.

Today, an individual with end-stage renal disease has prolonged life expectancy due in part to dialysis and kidney transplantation. Currently, about 10 percent of deaths associated with high blood pressure are due to kidney failure.

Many researchers contend that essential high blood pressure can be linked to a kidney that appears to be normal but has a diminished ability to rid the body of salt. (See the nearby sidebar "Is the kidney the source of most high blood pressure?") This scientific perspective is further supported by the fact that every society that consumes salt in large quantities has a high incidence of high blood pressure. Chapter 10 describes the close connection between salt and high blood pressure in greater detail.

Managing Malignant High Blood Pressure

Malignant high blood pressure (often found in smokers and in young African American males) affects about 1 percent of people with high blood pressure. It refers to severely high blood pressure (a diastolic reading often greater than 150 mm Hg) *and* severe complications including the following:

- Severe eye damage such as

  - *Papilledema* (swelling of the optic disc — where the nerve enters the eye from the brain)

  - *Exudates* (white spots from release of fluids that are opaque in front of the retina)

  - Bleeding from capillaries in the eye

  - Blindness

- Progressive damage to the brain that may first manifest itself as headaches (The individual may become confused and finally lapse into a coma.)

> ✔ Rapid development of partial or total loss of kidney function
>
> ✔ Nausea and vomiting
>
> ✔ Congestive heart failure

Dramatically elevated blood pressure isn't enough to make a malignant high blood pressure diagnosis, and people with the same high blood pressure reading may not have the condition. Several of the symptoms in the preceding list are necessary to make the diagnosis.

A doctor must treat malignant high blood pressure in a hospital setting because it's a medical emergency. The patient may not have had a diagnosis of high blood pressure in the past. He may appear confused, have heart failure, and have evidence of no remaining kidney function. (A physical exam should disclose the high blood pressure as well as the poor mental functioning.) When the doctor looks in the patient's eyes, she sees swelling of the optic disc, bleeding that can be small dots or flame-shaped hemorrhages, and spasm of the arteries within the eye.

The exact cause of malignant high blood pressure is unclear. Some possibilities include the following:

> ✔ **The direct result of poor blood pressure control.** The blood pressure is allowed to rise to this dangerous level.
>
> ✔ **The production of chemicals by damaged kidneys.** These chemicals further damage the kidney and cause contraction of blood vessels, thus raising the blood pressure.
>
> ✔ **Suppression of other chemicals that usually widen blood vessels.**

Causes of secondary high blood pressure (see Chapter 4), especially blocked kidney arteries *(renal artery stenosis)*, also trigger malignant high blood pressure in as many as one-third of the cases.

Understanding a kidney aneurysm

As *atherosclerosis* (the process by which cholesterol in the arteries leads to narrowing of the arteries and higher blood pressure; see Chapter 4) builds up in the body's blood vessels, it also affects the kidney arteries. But the wall of the kidney artery is weaker than a normal artery. So, under the influence of higher blood pressure, the wall bulges out until it forms an *aneurysm*, a thin sac that's filled with blood and is under high pressure. An aneurysm can rupture, leaking blood into the body. Unless the rupture is closed, the blood loss may lead to shock or death. A ruptured aneurysm must be considered when a patient with high blood pressure suddenly develops very low blood pressure.

In the days before 1950 or so, when treatment for high blood pressure wasn't available, the majority of patients with malignant high blood pressure were dead within six months. Now that effective treatment is available for lowering the pressure, the response to treatment depends on the amount of irreversible kidney damage:

- ✔ If the kidney damage is minimal, then more than 90 percent of patients are alive after five years.

- ✔ Among those with kidney damage, the survival is about 65 percent after five years.

   If these patients don't have a fatal heart attack, the eventual cause of death is end-stage renal disease (which I cover in the next section), particularly if their kidneys show signs of damage.

Coping with End-Stage Renal Disease

End-stage renal disease (ESRD), also known as *chronic renal failure,* is loss of at least 90 percent of kidney function. The kidneys can't perform their primary function — waste removal. Thus, waste and excess fluid (which normally pass through the urethra and out of the body) build up within the body. To continue living, the patient requires a kidney transplant or dialysis.

More than 500,000 people in the United States are being treated for ESRD, and the number rises 10 percent each year. In addition:

- ✔ About half of those with ESRD are men.

- ✔ About two-thirds are Caucasian and about one-third is African American.

- ✔ The largest group is between 45 and 64 years of age.

- ✔ Almost one-fifth of those with ESRD die each year.

- ✔ The cost of caring for people with ESRD is $30 billion each year.

High blood pressure, diabetes, and many other conditions that destroy the filtering nephrons (which I discuss earlier in this chapter) can lead to ESRD. However, individuals who are losing their kidney function are usually unaware of it until they begin to feel sick. In fact:

- ✔ Often, they don't start to feel sick until 90 percent of their kidneys' ability to get rid of toxins fails.

- ✔ High blood pressure, anemia, and bone disease can occur with about 70 percent of kidney function lost. But the individual may still be unaware of these abnormalities.

Efforts to reduce high blood pressure have greatly reduced the rate of heart disease (see Chapter 5) and brain attacks (see Chapter 7). But this result isn't the case for ESRD, probably because — throughout the world — high blood pressure isn't controlled sufficiently or long term. Whether high blood pressure is untreated or inadequately treated, the result is much the same: If the patient doesn't die of heart disease or a brain attack, ESRD will develop.

Currently the most common reasons for ESRD are diabetes (33 percent) and high blood pressure (25 percent); internal diseases of the kidney account for the rest.

The person with untreated ESRD is very ill. Symptoms affect the entire body and include the following:

- ✔ Fatigue and weakness
- ✔ Easy bruising
- ✔ Itchy skin that appears yellow-brown
- ✔ A metallic taste in the mouth
- ✔ Breath that smells of urine
- ✔ Shortness of breath (even while sitting still and more with minimal activity)
- ✔ Nausea and vomiting
- ✔ Weight loss
- ✔ Headache
- ✔ Impotency
- ✔ Frequent urination that interrupts sleep
- ✔ Cramping and spasms in the legs (especially at night while trying to sleep)
- ✔ Irritability
- ✔ Unconsciousness

These signs and symptoms subside after treatment begins. Whether the kidneys fail because of high blood pressure, diabetes, or some other cause, the kidney treatment at this stage is the same: dialysis or kidney transplantation.

The choices for the treatment of ESRD, detailed in the following sections, have their pluses and minuses. Ample financial resources are available for all the choices because the federal government as well as private insurance pay for most of the treatment cost. You needn't worry about paying for your care.

If your kidneys are failing and you take drugs for other conditions, the dosage of those drugs must be adjusted if they depend upon the urine for removal from the body. Discuss this with your doctor as you consider treatments for ESRD.

Lifesaving dialysis

If the kidneys fail, as in the case of ESRD, they can't filter out and eliminate the body's waste. As I describe in the earlier sidebar "Life before and after miracle drugs," an individual with ESRD and untreated high blood pressure can't expect to live much longer. In these cases, however, modern medicine's methods of waste removal, *peritoneal dialysis* or *hemodialysis,* can filter waste from the blood and rid the body of its nasty toxins. Of the 500,000 patients with ESRD in the United States, 350,000 are undergoing dialysis.

Peritoneal dialysis

If you have ESRD, you may need peritoneal dialysis, which takes advantage of the *peritoneum's* (the abdominal cavity's lining) filtering abilities. The peritoneum prevents the passage of larger elements of the blood, such as blood cells and protein, but allows the liquid part with all its dissolved substances to pass through.

Peritoneal dialysis consists of these steps:

1. A surgeon places a permanent catheter into the abdominal cavity.

2. A *dialysate,* a salt-and-sugar solution, is put into the abdominal cavity through the catheter.

3. Because of their high concentration, body wastes enter the dialysate solution.

4. The dialysate, along with the unwanted wastes, is drained out through the catheter.

Each cycle of putting in and removing dialysate is an *exchange.* Figure 6-4 shows a peritoneal dialysis.

Peritoneal dialysis is usually done at home and is much more successful with several exchanges per day instead of one. There are three types of peritoneal dialysis:

- ✓ **Continuous ambulatory peritoneal dialysis** uses gravity to fill and empty the abdomen. Usually the individual needs three to four daytime exchanges and one during sleep.

- ✓ **Continuous cycler-assisted peritoneal dialysis** uses a machine to fill and remove the dialysate from the abdomen, especially during the night to make the overnight dialysis more efficient. Three to five exchanges take place during sleep. Another, longer exchange takes place during the day using a higher concentration of sugar to promote more waste removal.

✔ **Nocturnal intermittent peritoneal dialysis** uses six or more nighttime exchanges with the cycler machine to avoid the daytime exchange. Because this technique isn't the most efficient, these patients usually have some remaining kidney function.

Testing the dialysate as well as the patient's blood and urine determines the efficiency of each exchange. Measurement of the waste products in these three fluids determines whether the patient needs more dialysis, more solution, a different amount of sugar in the solution, or all three adjustments.

Home peritoneal dialysis has several pros and cons. The advantages include the following:

✔ The patient is in control of the treatment, so scheduling around his lifestyle is easier.

✔ The patient doesn't have to travel to the hospital or dialysis center.

✔ Dietary restrictions are minimal with the exception of protein intake.

✔ By carrying supplies or shipping them ahead to the destination, the patient is able to travel.

✔ Particularly with nocturnal intermittent peritoneal dialysis, the patient may exercise.

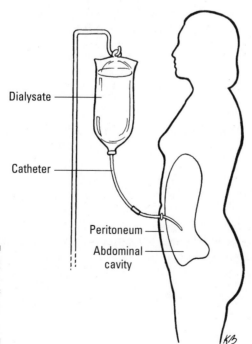

Figure 6-4:
The technique of peritoneal dialysis.

Dialysate

Catheter

Peritoneum

Abdominal cavity

The disadvantages include the following:

- Patients often fail to perform the dialysis, so they get sick.
- The patient must be trained to do the dialysis.
- Use of a cycler machine requires help from a partner.
- The dialysis bags and equipment require extra space in the home.
- *Peritonitis,* an infection of the peritoneal cavity, is a common complication.

Peritonitis raises body temperature. The abdomen may be tender and swollen, and the patient may be nauseated and vomiting. The dialysate becomes cloudy instead of clear, and bacteria may grow out from it.

If you notice these symptoms, see your doctor right away. Peritonitis is treatable and usually responds well to antibiotics. However, it sometimes recurs, and the bacteria infect the catheter. Then a new catheter is needed.

The success of peritoneal dialysis depends on:

- How much dialysate can be placed into the abdominal cavity
- How rapidly the wastes pass into the dialysate

Some people can't use peritoneal dialysis because their peritoneum doesn't allow sufficient rapid passage of body fluids. In this case, hemodialysis may be the preferred method of treating ESRD.

Other reasons why some people can't do peritoneal dialysis include:

- The presence of inflammatory bowel disease
- Inability to do self-care or lack of a caregiver
- Extensive prior abdominal surgery with many scars

Hemodialysis

During hemodialysis, your blood circulates through a *dialyzer* in the following steps:

1. A surgeon performs a minor operation in which an artery and a vein are connected to form an arteriovenous *fistula* (an abnormal connection) that allows for a large blood flow.

   The fistula heals in a month or so, and needles can then be placed in the artery (to deliver blood to the machine) and the vein (to return blood to the body).

2. The blood from the artery enters the dialyzer and passes through filters that mimic the glomerulus (see the earlier section "Focusing on

the filtering function"). Wastes are removed while normal body components are retained or returned to the blood.

3. The blood returns to the body through the needle into the vein.

Figure 6-5 shows a hemodialysis.

Hemodialysis usually lasts two to four hours, three times per week. Just as in peritoneal dialysis, the fluid produced by hemodialysis and the patient's blood can be tested to evaluate the adequacy of the treatment.

Hemodialysis, like peritoneal dialysis, has its share of advantages and disadvantages. Advantages include:

✔ It can be done at home, at a dialysis center, or within the hospital.

- Treatment at home allows you to set your own schedule as long as you follow your doctor's recommendations.

- Treatment at a hospital ensures that professional help is available in case it's needed. Also, because patients usually receive dialysis as a group, they often enjoy being in the company of other patients with similar problems.

✔ It takes considerably less time than peritoneal dialysis.

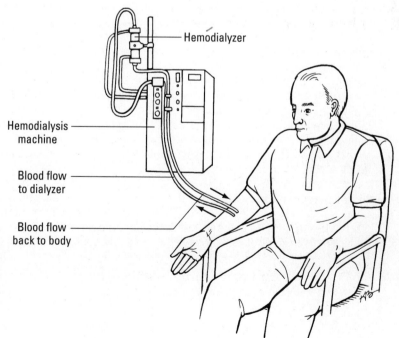

Hemodialyzer

Hemodialysis machine

Blood flow to dialyzer

Blood flow back to body

Figure 6-5: The technique of hemodialysis.

Disadvantages of hemodialysis include:

- ✔ Patients must follow a fairly careful diet and avoid fluids (depending on how much urine they're making), salt, foods that contain phosphorus (like milk, cheese, and chocolate), and foods that contain potassium (like citrus and tomatoes).

- ✔ Taking treatment away from the home requires regular trips to and from the hospital.

- ✔ The dialyzer and equipment take up plenty of space in the home.

- ✔ Patients must be trained to administer and monitor home hemodialysis. For example, they need to know how to clamp off the needles if bleeding occurs and must be vigilant about caring for the fistula to prevent infection.

Kidney transplantation

When possible, transplantation is the best answer to ESRD. You end up with a new, healthy kidney that performs like your *good* old kidneys. Of the 500,000 patients in the United States with ESRD, 150,000 have had kidney transplantation.

In kidney transplantation, you get a new kidney from a living related donor or from a donor who has recently passed away. If the kidney comes from a relative, you can have the surgery immediately. But for a kidney from a donor who has recently passed away, your name goes on a waiting list.

As shown in Figure 6-6, the kidney is placed in your lower abdomen during a surgery that takes about four hours. The failed kidneys are usually left in unless they're infected or causing high blood pressure. Arteries in the new kidney are attached to your arteries. As the figure shows, the ureter is transplanted to your bladder as well. The new kidney may take a few days or weeks to make urine. Hospitalization lasts another one to two weeks, and you can go back to work in four weeks.

Ninety percent of transplanted kidneys (whether from family members or unknown donors) still function after one year and eighty percent function after five years. On an average, kidneys from living donors survive 15 years, and kidneys from donors who have died last 10 years.

Before you can have a transplant, you must meet the following standards:

- ✔ You need to be well enough to withstand surgery and take the medications to prevent rejection.

- ✔ You are willing to take the medication without fail.

- ✔ You don't have other conditions that prevent successful transplantation (such as a cancer in the last two years, severe heart disease, or severe lung disease).

- ✔ You have a good support structure to help you.

Due to health reasons, only half of the patients on dialysis are appropriate for a transplant.

Kidney transplantation is a long-term solution with these significant advantages:

- ✔ Patients feel as normal as they did before they became sick.

- ✔ No dialysis is necessary as long as the kidney continues to function.

- ✔ Patients only need to follow a few dietary restrictions such as limiting foods high in fat, calories, and possibly sodium and potassium.

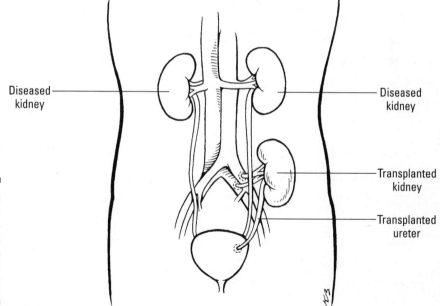

Figure 6-6:
Appearance
of a trans-
planted
kidney
in your
abdomen.

Diseased kidney

Diseased kidney

Transplanted kidney

Transplanted ureter

Like all the treatments, however, disadvantages exist:

- ✔ Transplantation requires major surgery.

- ✔ Few kidneys are available, so if the person has to wait for a donor, it may be a long wait, sometimes years. Meanwhile, dialysis is necessary.

- ✔ Some transplants fail, so a second transplant is needed.

- ✔ Patients must take drugs such as *immunosuppressants* for a lifetime to prevent the body from rejecting the transplanted kidney. These drugs have side effects such as the promotion of diabetes and the weakening of the immune system (making infection more likely).

- ✔ The drugs or rejection of the new kidney may be responsible for high blood pressure (present in up to 90 percent of transplant survivors), which can further damage the new kidney.

As of 2006, more than 65,000 people in the United States were awaiting transplantation. About 20,000 transplants are done each year, so the need for more surgeries is huge. The limiting factor is the supply of kidneys.

If you have healthy kidneys, consider placing a sticker on the back of your driver's license permitting the use of your kidneys as well as other organs if you die suddenly and unexpectedly. You will be giving the gift of life to two suffering people with your kidneys and the gift of sight to two others with your corneas.

If you are on the list for a transplant, be ready to go at a moment's notice. Have your bag packed and transportation available, and be prepared to stay in the area of the transplant center for up to four weeks. Check out the transplant center before you go by checking the database of the Scientific Registry of Transplant Recipients at www.ustransplant.org. Find out:

- ✔ The center's experience

- ✔ The survival of the center's transplants

- ✔ Other services (support groups and assistance with travel and housing)

You will be amazed at how many centers are available. For instance, California and Texas have 26 centers each that do kidney transplantation, and New York has 14. You will find a wide range of experience among those centers.

Chapter 7

Protecting Your Brain

● ●

In This Chapter

▶ Recognizing the different types of brain attacks

▶ Factoring in high blood pressure

▶ Knowing the risk factors and symptoms

▶ Testing, treating, and getting help for the brain attack survivor

● ●

*A*nnually, at least 5 million people throughout the world die from brain *attacks* (the term I prefer over *strokes* because the condition's similar to a heart attack), and 15 million more survive them. But brain attack survivors may live out the rest of their lives as dependents — unable to speak coherently and/or confined to a wheelchair because of the paralysis that results.

A brain attack isn't necessarily a disease of the elderly; 28 percent of the new cases are people under age 65. In the United States, 700,000 people have brain attacks each year and 162,000 die. Seventy percent of those who survive live without the assistance of others, but 30 percent are permanently disabled. Four million brain attack survivors in the United States have some degree of disability. In Japan, the incidence of brain attacks was in decline for many years, but now it's rising. In Eastern Europe and countries of the Russian Federation, the incidence is also rising, and many more brain attacks are fatal there as compared to more advanced areas like the United States, Canada, and Western Europe.

A *brain attack,* also known as a *cerebrovascular accident,* occurs when blood flow to a part of the brain is cut off. Depending on the severity of the attack, victims often suffer from impaired vision and speech, convulsions, paralysis, and coma. The higher the blood pressure, the greater the likelihood of a brain attack.

Brain attacks don't favor any particular group such as the poor or the rich, the famous, or the unknown. Perhaps one of the most famous people to suffer a brain attack was United States President Franklin Delano Roosevelt. In 1945, as World War II was coming to a close, President Roosevelt died within a few hours of a brain attack at the age of 63 after years of poorly treated high blood pressure. The famous nineteenth-century French bacteriologist, Louis Pasteur, on the other hand, suffered a brain attack at age 46 that left him paralyzed on the left side. Yet Pasteur — making medical history and discovering, among other findings, several bacteria that are responsible for the spread of infectious disease — did his best work during the next 25 years of his life.

In this chapter, I explain the causes of brain attacks, the warning signs that predict a brain attack, and signs that a brain attack is taking place. I also cover the value of early diagnosis and treatment and how to work with a brain attack survivor who needs rehabilitation. Make sure you have a handle on all the information in this chapter so this devastating complication never makes your life miserable. For even more information, check out *Stroke For Dummies* by John R. Marler (Wiley).

I separate my discussion of the brain from the heart (see Chapter 5) and the kidneys (see Chapter 6), but that doesn't mean a person develops brain damage from high blood pressure separate from heart disease or kidney failure. High blood pressure — the silent killer — tends to work its way on various parts of the body simultaneously. As a result, you may discover you have problems in all three areas at the same time.

Understanding the Causes of Brain Attacks

The belief that brain attacks were random events like bolts of lightning persisted into the twentieth century along with the term *apoplexy,* coming from a Greek word meaning *to be thunderstruck.* So folks back then used *apoplexy* to refer to a brain attack. Considered an unpreventable accident, a brain attack was also termed *cerebrovascular accident.* This explanation is clearly not the case, however.

Brain attacks, perhaps more than heart attacks and kidney failure, are preventable.

Progress in the treatment of high blood pressure between 1960 and 1990 made this complication of high blood pressure less common. More recently, however, the prevention of brain attacks has slowed down as a result of both diminished awareness and inadequate treatment. Even with the reduction in the incidence of brain attacks, it remains the third leading cause of death after heart attacks and cancer.

Although the correlation between high blood pressure and brain attacks is unmistakable (see the later section "Avoiding Brain Attacks by Reducing High Blood Pressure" for details), brain attacks come about in a variety of ways: from atherosclerosis, a cerebral embolus, or a brain hemorrhage.

Atherosclerosis

Just as *atherosclerosis* (damage to the inside of arteries caused by cholesterol deposits) can affect the arteries of the heart (see Chapter 5), it can also affect the arteries leading into and within the brain. About 60 percent of all brain attacks result from atherosclerosis, which is characterized by fatty deposits on the inner walls of the arteries. As a result, blood flow to critical parts of the brain is diminished. If the blood flow ceases entirely, a brain attack may occur.

The blood supply to the brain has multiple sources. (Figure 7-1 shows the unique circulation of blood in the brain.) Left and right *cerebral* arteries entering the skull in the front of the brain combine with left and right *vertebral* arteries entering the skull in the back of the brain to produce a circle of blood supply called the *circle of Willis* at the base of the brain. Other arteries that make up the circle are also shown in the figure. If one of the arteries is blocked, blood from the other arteries can fill the circle and provide blood to all areas of the brain. But the brain tissue dies when several sources of blood are blocked and the circulation isn't reopened within three hours.

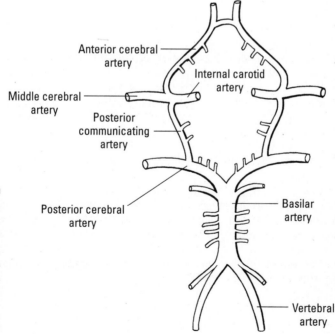

Anterior cerebral artery

Internal carotid artery

Middle cerebral artery

Posterior communicating artery

Posterior cerebral artery

Basilar artery

Vertebral artery

Figure 7-1: The unique joining of separate blood vessels form the circle of Willis.

Cerebral embolus

Approximately 25 percent of brain attacks are due to cerebral emboli.
A *cerebral embolus* is a blood clot (a solid mass of blood cells, protein, and
other blood substances) or solid tissue that breaks off from an *atherosclerotic
plaque* (an irregularity inside the artery; the end result of a cholesterol
deposit) and travels into the brain. The bloodstream carries the atherosclerotic plaque particle from its site of origin, often a large artery in the neck,
into the arteries of the brain, where it becomes wedged and then cuts off
circulation.

Blood clots usually come from the left atrium of the heart in the following
steps:

1. The heart loses its regular beating pattern and gives way to *atrial
   fibrillation* (uncoordinated twitching movements).

2. The heart's left atrium fails to completely empty its blood.

3. The pool of blood that remains forms clots that can break off and travel
   via the bloodstream into the arteries of the brain.

Brain hemorrhage

Brain hemorrhage — bleeding within the brain or between the skull and the
brain — accounts for the remaining 15 percent of brain attacks. Of these
attacks, two-thirds occur within the brain. As a result of high blood pressure
or other diseases, the muscular wall of the artery may weaken and form one
or more *aneurysms* (little pouches). Looking like a balloon attached to the
artery, an aneurysm can burst and bleed into the brain. However, because
the brain doesn't have extra space to make room for the extra blood, brain
tissue is squeezed and may die. ***Note:*** Bleeding within the brain can also
occur as a result of trauma to the head.

The other one-third of brain hemorrhages occur outside the brain in the
subarachnoid space — the thin separation between the inside of your bony skull
and the outside of your brain's fleshy gray matter. Bleeding within this space
usually results from an aneurysm that forms inside the skull but outside the
brain. If the aneurysm ruptures, the blood flows around the brain, causing
increased pressure and a severe headache that's often accompanied by
vomiting.

Avoiding Brain Attacks by Reducing High Blood Pressure

High blood pressure is the most important factor in the development of a brain attack, and its control can prevent such an attack. High blood pressure may hasten a brain attack by

- Speeding up the development of atherosclerosis
- Promoting the thickening of the middle layer of the arteries (This causes narrowing of the arteries and reduced blood flow into the brain.)
- Damaging small arteries to the point that they collapse
- Increasing the size of an aneurysm in the brain
- Causing thinning of the aneurysm to the point of rupture and hemorrhage
- Causing formation of aneurysms that rupture in the subarachnoid space to produce a subarachnoid hemorrhage

Many clinical trials have shown that reduction of blood pressure reduces the incidence of brain attacks, no matter how high the initial blood pressure or how old the patient. All types of brain attacks are reduced, from those caused by clots to those caused by hemorrhage. Part III is full of useful information on reducing high blood pressure.

Surveying Additional Predisposing Conditions

In addition to high blood pressure (the number-one contributor), other predisposing conditions play an important role in brain attacks. These risk factors are divided into what you *can't* control and what you *can* control. Obviously, you want to direct all your emphasis and energy towards factors that you can change. And if you have one or more unchangeable conditions, you must work even harder to minimize those controllable factors.

The hand you're dealt: Uncontrolled factors

You're born with most of these uncontrollable risk factors for a brain attack:

- ✔ **Age:** The older you get, the more you're at risk.

- ✔ **Sex:** At any age, brain attacks tend to occur more often among men than women, but women are more likely to die from their brain attack than men are.

- ✔ **Family history:** If one or more of your parents and grandparents had a brain attack, then you're at risk.

- ✔ **History of brain attack:** If you're a brain attack survivor, then you're at risk for another one.

The hand you play: Risk factors you control

With some risk factors you can *really* make a difference. (Part III shows you how.) The risk factors that are well within your power to change are

- ✔ **Alcoholic drinks:** Drinking more than two glasses of wine, hard liquor, or beer for men or one glass for women each night may contribute to a brain attack.

- ✔ **Arteriosclerosis:** This disease can be treated, and the arteries to the brain reopened. See Chapter 5 for more details.

- ✔ **Atrial fibrillation:** The irregular rhythm of the heartbeat associated with clots that block brain arteries can be brought under control with the help of the right treatment. Ask your doctor.

- ✔ **Diabetes:** The high blood glucose of uncontrolled diabetes associated with high blood pressure and high cholesterol can be brought under control. Check out my book *Diabetes For Dummies,* 2nd Edition (Wiley) for more information.

- ✔ **Excess weight and obesity:** Even if you're only ten pounds overweight, that excess ten pounds contributes to high blood pressure and diabetes. However, dieting and exercising can reduce your weight.

- ✔ **High blood cholesterol:** Even without diabetes, cholesterol increases the risk of a brain attack. Diet, exercise, and medications, if necessary, can control this factor.

✔ **Illegal drugs:** Using illegal drugs such as amphetamine, ecstasy, and cocaine increases blood pressure and your chances of a brain attack.

✔ **Lack of exercise:** A sedentary lifestyle predisposes you to a brain attack, but exercise can drastically decrease your chances of having a brain attack.

✔ **Tobacco:** Smoking cigarettes or cigars or chewing tobacco reduces oxygen in the blood and damages the walls of the blood vessels. Conversely, kicking your tobacco habit oxygenates the blood and decreases the likelihood of damaged blood vessels.

✔ **Transient ischemic attack (TIA):** This is a milder form of brain attack, and TIA symptoms are always temporary. (See the "Moving Fast When You See Symptoms of a Brain Attack" section later in this chapter.) Drugs can reduce the incidence of these attacks.

If you keep these risk factors under control, you're sure to decrease the likelihood of a disabling brain attack.

Funduscopic examination minus the fun

When a doctor looks into your eyes with an ophthalmoscope (called a *funduscopic exam*), he's observing the one area of the brain that can be seen directly. High blood pressure causes changes in the blood vessels of your eyes that are similar to the changes it causes in small blood vessels in the brain.

The earliest change that the doctor sees with the ophthalmoscope is a narrowing of the arteries: The artery walls thicken, and although blood may still flow, the column of blood is not visible and the artery looks like a silver wire. As the arteries thicken, nearby veins are also compressed, and *arteriovenous* (AV) *nicking* (a compression of a vein where the artery crosses it) appears.

Your physician may see other changes in your eyes due to high blood pressure with his ophthalmoscope:

✔ The eye's major central retinal vein, which carries blood away from the retina (the tissue that acts as a screen for sight), can close. Then vision is lost in that eye, and the back of the eye appears to be bleeding.

✔ As blood flow fails, areas of the retina die, leaving a white, patchy appearance (called *cotton wool spots*).

✔ Appearing as sacs attached to arteries, aneurysms can form in the arteries of the eyes just as elsewhere in the brain due to the high blood pressure. They rarely cause hemorrhage within the eye, but if they do, it may be necessary to clot them with laser treatment.

✔ Hemorrhaging from the retina's arteries produces a flame-shaped area in the retina — a sign of *malignant* or *accelerated* (out-of-control) high blood pressure (Chapter 6 discusses this condition).

Working some miracles with preventive drugs

If you're at high risk to have a stroke because you previously had one or had a TIA or because you have atrial fibrillation or narrowing of the *carotid* arteries (the main arteries arising from the aorta that provide blood to the brain), a number of drugs can lower the risk. The most valuable are as follows:

- **Aspirin, a drug that prevents platelets in the blood from forming a clot:** If you have a TIA, aspirin may reduce your risk of a stroke by 30 percent. You should use no more than a baby aspirin (81 milligrams) daily, but check with your doctor.

- **Clopidogrel (Plavix), an antiplatelet drug:** It doesn't cause the gastrointestinal bleeding of aspirin, but its reduction of stroke risk is similar to aspirin's.

- **Dipyridamole plus Aspirin (Aggrenox):** This drug helps prevent a second stroke for people who have already had one but causes gastrointestinal bleeding more often than aspirin.

- **Anticoagulants such as warfarin (Coumadin):** These drugs prevent formation of clots but run the risk of excessive bleeding. They must be monitored with blood tests, which are inconvenient.

Interestingly, a study in the January 2007 *Archives of Internal Medicine* indicates that combining aspirin and oral anticoagulants like warfarin provides no better protection than aspirin alone and runs the risk of much increased major bleeding.

Moving Fast When You See Symptoms of a Brain Attack

The symptoms of an impending brain attack come on suddenly. Don't waste a minute getting to a hospital. You may prevent much of the damage if you receive treatment within the first three hours. If you experience any of the following symptoms or see another individual displaying one or all of them, call an ambulance!

- Sudden blurred or decreased vision in one or both eyes
- Numbness, weakness, or paralysis of the face, arm, or leg on one or both sides of the body
- Difficulty speaking or understanding
- Sudden dizziness, loss of balance, or an unexplained fall

✔ Nausea, vomiting, or difficulty swallowing

✔ Sudden headache or change in the pattern of headaches

If these symptoms last 5 to 20 minutes (and never more than 24 hours), the condition is a TIA. It's usually the result of

✔ Completely blocked arteries that are rapidly reopened by certain chemicals in the blood or the force of the blood pressure

✔ Small *emboli* (see the earlier section "Cerebral embolus") that briefly interrupt blood flow. The emboli can be dissolved by drugs or bypassed by using a blood vessel or artificial tube to go around the blockage.

One-third of TIA victims eventually suffer a severe brain attack with permanent symptoms, but the other two-thirds don't. TIAs must be taken seriously, and the patient needs a doctor's evaluation to see whether the cause is an atherosclerotic plaque in an artery or atrial fibrillation. The doctor can bypass the plaque surgically or provide anticoagulants to prevent clotting from atrial fibrillation.

Capturing Brain Function on Film

The brain is specialized; each area performs certain functions. When a brain attack occurs, the doctor pinpoints the damaged part of the brain to first localize the probable blocked or bleeding artery and then determine whether treatment is feasible. Figure 7-2 shows the location of the various functions.

As you can see, loss of blood supply to specific areas of the brain can result in the loss of a specific function and consequent signs and symptoms (see the previous section for a list of these signs). Because the right side of the brain controls the left side of the body, and because the nerves cross over, careful *mapping* of the loss of function (noting the nerves that correspond) can determine the area of the brain that's damaged. For example, paralysis of the left leg means that the right brain leg control area is knocked out.

Some functions like memory, however, are controlled by only one side of the brain. If the brain attack affects the right side of the brain, for example, the victim may experience some of the following symptoms in addition to weakness or paralysis on the left side of his body:

✔ Tendency to be impulsive or disorganized

✔ Lack of coordination and tendency to fall

✔ Inability to remember

✔ Lack of insight and judgment

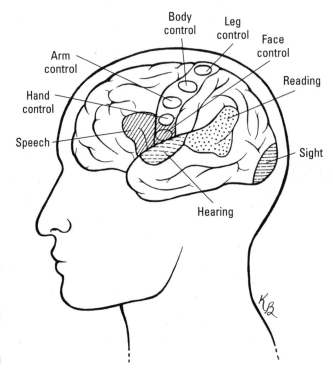

Figure 7-2:
Sites in the
brain that
control body
functions.

If the brain attack occurs on the left side of your brain, you may experience some difficulty communicating in addition to right-sided weakness or paralysis.

Although specific sites in the brain affect corresponding bodily functions, scientists don't fully understand and can't exactly locate which arteries affect that specific brain site because of the overabundance of cross circulation in the brain. As a result, mapping of function loss can determine the *affected* area, but determining the *source* of the impairment (like an aneurysm within an artery that feeds the brain) may be extremely difficult.

Other symptoms that aren't particular to one side of the body may follow a brain attack. For example, the survivor may not see or think as she did before; her perceptions are altered. As a result, she may be depressed or suffer mood swings — suddenly bursting into laughter for no apparent reason. In another instance, one side of the body is weaker and vision on that side is poorer. The individual may lose awareness of that side of her body and tend to bump into objects with that side.

The doctor may need to perform various sophisticated tests to clarify where the damage has occurred and why. The following list describes a few of the tests your doctor may perform:

✔ **Computerized axial tomography (CAT scan)** or **magnetic resonance imaging (MRI)** can

- • Pinpoint the location of dead brain cells

- • Examine minute areas of the brain

- • Differentiate between a TIA and a hemorrhage

In addition, the MRI can look for aneurysms and malformations that can eventually cause hemorrhage in the arteries and veins.

The patient's head is placed within a circular machine that takes X-rays from different angles. It's painless!

✔ **Digital subtraction angiographies (DSA)** take X-rays after dye has been injected directly into the brain's circulation. DSA can pinpoint the brain's blood vessels that are prohibiting normal circulation of the blood.

✔ **Doppler ultrasound** tests evaluate blood flow in an artery. Sound waves are directed to the artery (usually in the neck in this case) to indicate whether blood is flowing slowly or normally.

✔ **Electroencephalograms (EEG)** test electrical activity in the brain to

- • Indicate whether the brain is functioning and, if so, where.

- • Determine whether an unconscious person is brain dead after a brain attack so a ventilator (to help the victim breathe) can be continued or disconnected.

In this painless procedure, electrodes are directly applied to the scalp surface.

Multiplying the Treatments for Brain Attacks

When a brain attack occurs, usually the *ischemic core* (area of restricted blood supply) suffers a permanent loss of brain cells. The *ischemic penumbra* (the larger area around that core) is still alive and can be saved with quick action using a *tissue plasminogen activator* (tPA, brand name Activase) or another clot-dissolving drug to break up any clot or obstruction to the flow of blood. This drug must be used within the first three hours after the brain attack to really benefit the brain and prevent more tissue loss.

Obviously, the doctor can't use a tPA in a hemorrhagic brain attack (see the earlier section "Brain hemorrhage") because it doesn't involve blood clots. Unfortunately, hemorrhage is an occasional side effect of tPAs and can then bring on another brain attack.

Patients who have had a brain attack use the same drugs to prevent future attacks (I discuss these drugs earlier in this chapter):

- ✔ **Aspirin** to prevent further attacks if you've had a TIA
- ✔ **Warfarin** for

  - Frequent and unstable TIAs

  - Atrial fibrillation (see the "Cerebral embolus" section earlier in this chapter for more about this condition)

In addition to drugs, the following procedures are possible:

- ✔ **Clipping** or tying off a bleeding aneurysm that's the source of the brain attack may stop the bleeding and prevent it from rupturing. The decision to perform this procedure depends on the location of the aneurysm. It may not be approachable without damaging important brain tissue.
- ✔ **Endarterectomies** can remove an obstruction, especially in the carotid arteries (the arteries outside the brain). During this surgery, the doctor opens the neck where the artery is blocked and removes the blockage. *Note:* Even if surgery successfully repairs one blood vessel, it may not cure the problem because the brain's blood supply comes from so many blood vessels; others may also be obstructed.
- ✔ **Merci Retrieval System** is a new technique to treat ischemic brain attacks due to blockage. The doctor threads a catheter into the obstructed blood vessel, grabs the clot with the Merci device at the end of the catheter, and then removes the clot through the catheter. The procedure works about half the time, especially for larger clots.

- ✔ **Stents** can be used in carotid artery blockage just as they are in coronary artery blockage (see Chapter 5 for information). So far, though, studies haven't determined whether carotid endarterectomy or stenting is the better procedure.

Making Your Way Back through Rehabilitation

Preventing a brain attack is so much better than having to deal with the consequences of a brain attack. Nevertheless, millions of people throughout the world have suffered brain attacks, and an enormous amount of resources is available for brain attack survivors. The following sections provide some insights into what the brain attack victim can expect after the attack and how to get help. The Internet can be a great resource, and I offer some of its most useful sites.

Current methods of treatment are excellent, and resources are so great that the vast majority of people who have suffered a brain attack can return to some level of satisfactory function in the long term.

Regaining movement following a brain attack

Most people who have had a brain attack have trouble swallowing initially because the swallowing muscles and the mouth have been affected. They must often be supported with intravenous feeding until they can swallow without the food going into the trachea, the tube leading into the lungs.

It may take a month after the brain attack to determine how much function is going to return and what retraining has to take place. However, rehabilitation begins within 24 hours of a stroke if the patient is stable enough. The patient is encouraged to move and change position often, from lying in bed to sitting to standing and walking if possible. If limbs are paralyzed, the nurse or physical therapist moves the limbs passively.

As time passes, therapists help the patient to perform the activities of daily living: bathing, shaving, brushing teeth, combing hair, and using the toilet. When the patient starts regaining these skills, he begins to have confidence that his life isn't over and that he may be able to function independently after all.

Checking out rehabilitation locations

The location and goals of rehabilitation depend on the limitations of the brain attack survivor. Several rehabilitation choices are available:

- ✔ **In-home therapy:** Sometimes, the physical therapist comes to a person's home because the brain attack survivor can live at home but can't be transported to the hospital. This is also an opportunity for the therapist to inspect the home and offer suggestions that protect the patient from accidents and make activities of daily living more efficient.

- ✔ **Inpatient rehabilitation unit:** Rehabilitation can take place at the hospital if the survivor is immobile and unable to take care of himself. The unit's staff carefully analyzes the survivor's level of function and sets clear goals for restoration. For several hours daily, six days a week, the patient works with physical therapists, doctors, specialized nurses, and the best equipment to regain his self-sufficiency.

✔ **Nursing facility:** Brain attack survivors who can't go home alone but also don't need the inpatient rehabilitation unit can go to a nursing facility. *Skilled nursing facilities* perform rehabilitation, and a *nursing home* provides mostly food and shelter along with medications as needed.

✔ **Outpatient rehabilitation unit:** After the survivor can move around fairly well (or if the physical disabilities don't prevent a satisfactory life outside the hospital), he goes to an outpatient unit and returns home after each treatment. The unit may be at the hospital with the same doctors, nurses, and other specialists, but treatment doesn't take place on a daily basis. The program depends on the survivor's needs.

Meeting rehabilitation specialists

A *physiatrist* (specializing in physical medicine and rehabilitation) completely evaluates the patient and determines the patient's physical limitations. With the help of the other rehabilitation specialists, she draws up a plan of action including goals and time frames. The following list includes the titles and responsibilities of other rehabilitation specialists:

✔ **Occupational therapist:** Teaches the skills needed to perform physical work, whether it's cleaning the house, gardening, painting, or other crafts. They teach patients how to perform tasks with one hand that normally require two hands, for example, and how to make the home safe and more efficient.

✔ **Physical therapist:** Helps the patient regain muscular movement and strength in the affected limbs *and* use the unaffected limbs to compensate for loss of function. To overcome the patient's lack of awareness of affected limbs, therapists use *selective sensory stimulation,* a technique that stimulates the limbs.

✔ **Rehabilitation nurse:** Trains the brain attack patient to perform the activities of daily living including transferring from bed to chair, bathing, and controlling urination if incontinence is a problem.

✔ **Speech-language pathologist:** Helps patients who've developed *aphasia* (inability to speak properly after a brain attack) to regain speech. The pathologist also evaluates swallowing, determines the cause of the disability, and then provides techniques to correct the problem.

✔ **Vocational therapist:** Helps the patient to regain useful work using the patient's greatest strengths. Therapists work as job counselors for patients, informing them of their rights as disabled workers and helping them find suitable work that accommodates their residual limitations.

Sex after a brain attack

You don't have to give up sex after a brain attack because it doesn't increase the risk of another brain attack. After you've stabilized, you can have sexual relations consistent with whatever limitations the brain attack has imposed. Sex after a brain attack is most pleasurable when the same conditions are present as before a brain attack: the right partner, the right environment, and the right feelings.

Finding help after a brain attack

Resources for the person who has suffered a brain attack are plentiful. Most resources are on the Internet, but I also provide addresses so you can get information through the mail as well.

With these resources and the amazing number of links that their Web sites point to, you should get an answer to any question. Someone else who has had the same experience or has asked the same question is always out there.

- ✔ **American Stroke Association** is a subdivision of the American Heart Association. It offers many publications on the causes, natural history, and treatments of brain attacks as well as publications about high blood pressure. The association also offers *Stroke Connection Magazine* with timely articles on all aspects of brain attacks.

  Web site: www.strokeassociation.org

  Mailing address: American Stroke Association, 7272 Greenville Avenue, Dallas, TX 75231

  Phone: 888-478-7653 (888-4-STROKE); 800-553-6321

  Registry of over 2,000 stroke support groups

  Phone: 888-478-7653

- ✔ **Family Caregiver Alliance** was the first organization to offer help to people caring for a loved one. It offers everything you need to know about caregiving for patients with brain attacks and many other medical conditions.

  Web site: www.caregiver.org

  Mailing address: Family Caregiver Alliance, 180 Montgomery Street, Suite 1100, San Francisco, CA 94104

  Phone: 800-445-8106

✔ **The National Aphasia Association** promotes public education, research, rehabilitation, and support services to assist people with aphasia and their families. It sells educational gifts and helps to form support groups for aphasia patients. The Web site is packed with useful information and many personal accounts of a brain attack and the aphasia that followed; its links on aphasia make the site invaluable.

Web site: `aphasia.org`

Mailing address: The National Aphasia Association, 350 Seventh Avenue, Suite 902, New York, NY 10001

Phone: 800-922-4622

✔ **National Institute of Neurological Disorders and Stroke (NINDS)** has a huge database on every aspect of brain attacks. Of great interest are the studies that patients can enter such as "Observational Learning in Stroke Patients" and "Vitamin Therapy for Prevention of Strokes."

Web site: `www.ninds.nih.gov`; the site has numerous publications and fact sheets that you can copy or order.

Mailing address: NIH Neurological Institute, P.O. Box 5801, Bethesda, MD 20824

Phone: 800-352-9424

✔ **National Rehabilitation Information Center** is funded by the federal government to serve anyone on topics concerning rehabilitation. Their database is vast and their links to more rehabilitation information are outstanding.

Web site: `www.naric.com`

Mailing address: National Rehabilitation Information Center, 8201 Corporate Drive, Suite 600, Landover, MD 20785

Phone: 800-346-2742

✔ **National Stroke Association** calls itself the *voice for stroke,* and its mission is "to reduce the incidence and impact of this life-threatening medical condition." The association offers publications on the cause, prevention, and treatment of a brain attack and on rehabilitation after a brain attack.

Web site: `www.stroke.org`

Mailing address: National Stroke Association, 9707 East Easter Lane, Centennial, CO 80112

Phone: 800-787-6537 (800-STROKES)

✔ **Strokes Clubs International** offers help and experience *from* people with brain attacks *to* people with brain attacks.

Mailing address: Strokes Clubs International, 805 12th Street, Galveston, TX 77550

Phone: 409-762-1022

Part III

Treating (Or Preventing) High Blood Pressure

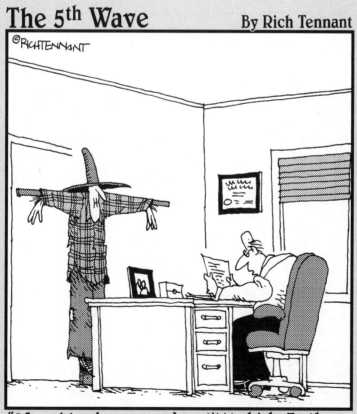

The 5th Wave   By Rich Tennant

"Your blood pressure's a little high. Is there any way you can incorporate some aerobic activity into your daily schedule?"

In this part . . .

Fortunately, you can treat (or prevent) high blood pressure in multiple ways so it never damages you. Starting with lifestyle changes and ending with drugs (only if absolutely necessary), this part gives you all the necessary tools. No one need ever suffer a heart attack, a brain attack, or kidney failure as a result of high blood pressure.

Chapter 8

Developing a Successful Treatment Plan

*T*wo truths should motivate you to create a successful treatment plan for your high blood pressure:

- ✔ High blood pressure must be brought under control to prevent the devastating consequences of uncontrolled high blood pressure — heart, kidney, and brain damage (I cover these in Part II).

- ✔ High blood pressure can be brought under control in any patient using the tools that are currently available.

Surprisingly, the progress in people's awareness, amounts of treatment, and amounts of successful treatment of high blood pressure in the last few decades has been little.

- ✔ In the United States in the 1980s, 73 percent of the population with high blood pressure was aware of their condition, but in the first decade of the twenty-first century, this number has dropped to 70 percent.

- ✔ In the 1980s, 55 percent of the people with high blood pressure were being treated, but that number has gone up only 4 percent in recent years.

- ✔ Of those treated in the 1980s, 29 percent were under control. In recent years the figure is 34 percent.

These figures mean almost a third of the people with high blood pressure don't know they have it, two-fifths of the people who *do* know it aren't receiving treatment, and two-thirds of patients receiving treatment are not meeting their goals.

This performance is unacceptable. Other countries are doing no better and are generally worse. You and your physician are the ones who can turn this around. Start right now — sit down and write an outline for the elements of a successful treatment plan. This chapter can help you.

Achieving Your Treatment Goal

You need a goal to know where you're going. Your particular goal depends on your present blood pressure.

- ✔ If you have normal blood pressure (less than 120/80 mm Hg), you want to keep it normal.

- ✔ If you already have *prehypertension* (see Chapter 2 for an explanation of this term) or high blood pressure, you want to lower it into the normal range and keep it there.

- ✔ If you already have complications of high blood pressure, you want to prevent them from progressing and even reverse them if possible.

Damage due to high blood pressure is continuous. *Target-organ damage* (damage to organs of the body from high blood pressure) doesn't start suddenly at 120/80 mm Hg; it creeps up on you slowly. As a result, people on the high side of *normal* blood pressure have a greater chance of suffering complications associated with their blood pressure than people on the low side of normal blood pressure, and people in the pre-hypertension range average more medical complications than those in the normal range.

Table 8-1 shows what category your blood pressure falls into and the recommended follow-up. (Also, see the table on blood pressure classifications in Chapter 2.)

If you already have diabetes mellitus or kidney disease and your reading is greater than 130/80, you have stage 1 high blood pressure.

Table 8-1	Recommended Follow-up Based on Initial Blood Pressure Measurements		
Category	Systolic (mm Hg)	Diastolic (mm Hg)	Follow-up by physician
Normal	Less than 120	Less than 80	Recheck in 2 years
Prehypertension	120–139	80–89	Recheck in 1 year; give lifestyle advice
Stage 1 HBP	140–159	90–99	Confirm in 2 months; use one blood pressure medication plus lifestyle advice if still present
Stage 2 HBP	Greater than or equal to 160	Greater than or equal to 100	Evaluate/refer to care within 1 month; use two BP medications plus lifestyle advice

Courtesy of The National Heart, Lung and Blood Institute of the National Institutes of Health in the Seventh Report of the Joint National Committee on Detection, Evaluation, and Treatment of High Blood Pressure (2003)

The National Heart, Lung and Blood Institute of the National Institutes of Health in the Seventh Report of the Joint National Committee (JNC 7) on Detection, Evaluation, and Treatment of High Blood Pressure (2003) provides a list of important risk factors for high blood pressure (see Chapter 3 for more details). The risk factors are

✔ Age (older than 55 for men, 65 for women)

✔ Diabetes

✔ Family history of heart disease

✔ High blood cholesterol

✔ *Microalbuminuria* (the presence of more than 30 but less than 300 milligrams of albumin in the urine in 24 hours)

✔ Obesity

✔ Physical inactivity

✔ Smoking

A new recommendation of the JNC 7 is that every patient with stage 1 or stage 2 high blood pressure — with or without the previous list of risk factors — should be treated. The risk factors (also called *compelling indications* for treatment) only increase the *urgency* of treatment.

JNC 7 offers a treatment *algorithm* (a series of logical steps) to bring the blood pressure to normal:

1. If you have prehypertension, modify your lifestyle.

2. If high blood pressure is present, use lifestyle modifications (which I discuss later in this chapter).

3. If lifestyle modification is unsuccessful, begin drugs (see Chapter 13 for full details on blood pressure medication).

   • If no compelling indications are present with stage 1 high blood pressure, most people can begin with thiazide diuretics.

   • If no compelling indications are present with stage 2 high blood pressure, use two drugs, a thiazide diuretic, and another class of drugs.

   • If compelling indications exist — regardless of the stage — use a specific drug for the indication plus other classes of drugs.

4. If blood pressure goals are still not achieved, increase dosages of the drugs and add other drugs until blood pressure is under control.

You can take these measures right now:

✔ Determine what your blood pressure is with the help of your physician.

✔ Discuss your risk factors and how they affect your treatment.

✔ Use the doctor's expertise to formulate a plan that reverses your reversible risk factors and lowers your blood pressure.

A few examples from my practice can help you to understand the road ahead.

✔ Joe Chang is a 43-year-old Chinese American who came to me because his blood pressure was elevated. Examining him, I determined that he was 5 feet and 5 inches tall and weighed 180 pounds. He didn't have diabetes or any other risk factor. He hadn't followed a diet and didn't exercise. On several different occasions, I found that his blood pressure was about 144/95 mm Hg. Based on the table of treatment strategies, I told him to begin a program of diet and exercise and referred him to a dietitian. Three months later, he had lost ten pounds and was exercising regularly. His blood pressure had fallen to 138/86 mm Hg. He has continued the program and lost an additional ten pounds with continued good blood pressure control.

✔ Elaine David, a 38-year-old mother of two children, has diabetes. I followed her through her two uncomplicated pregnancies. She weighs 160 pounds and is 5 feet 3 inches tall. Recently, her blood pressure has measured 165/98 mm Hg. She doesn't have any other risk factors (see the earlier list in this section). Elaine needed to lose weight, exercise more, reduce her salt intake, and get on drug treatment. I placed her on hydrochlorothiazide 12.5 milligrams daily; when her blood pressure was still over 140/90 mm Hg, I added enalapril. On this treatment, plus weight loss and exercise, her blood pressure is now 132/80 mm Hg and she feels well.

✔ Phil Sweeney is a 62-year-old new patient. His weight was appropriate for his height. His blood pressure, however, was 175/105 mm Hg, and he had evidence of eye damage due to high blood pressure as well as an enlarged heart. On this basis, I started him on two medications in view of his stage 2 high blood pressure, asked him to continue his good diet with some salt reduction, and asked him to do a little more exercise. His response has been gratifying — a reduction in the size of his heart and a drop in his blood pressure to 136/88 mm Hg. He has done some meditation as well, which seems to help. He tells me he feels like a new man.

Outlining Lifestyle Modifications

Chapters 9 through 12 of this book discuss suggested lifestyle changes in detail. In this section, I outline these changes so you can see the general approach to high blood pressure treatment. (See Chapter 13 for a complete discussion of treating high blood pressure with medication.) Just for laughs . . . and your good health, I also explain how tickling your funny bone can help your blood pressure drop.

Altering your lifestyle for the better

The JNC 7 on Detection, Evaluation and Treatment of High Blood Pressure recommends the following lifestyle modifications:

✔ Reduce saturated fat and cholesterol in your diet (Chapter 9)

✔ Maintain adequate potassium, calcium, and magnesium in your diet (Chapters 9 and 10)

✔ Reduce salt in your diet (Chapters 9 and 10)

✔ Lose weight (Chapters 9 and 12)

✔ Limit alcohol intake (Chapter 11)

✔ Stop smoking or chewing tobacco (Chapter 11)

✔ Increase physical activity (Chapter 12)

Starting with small, easy changes

The preceding list contains no surprises, with the possible exception of maintaining potassium, calcium, and magnesium. Doctors have known for years that these minerals help to lower blood pressure. So, you're wise to get sufficient quantities of them in your diet. These suggestions can help:

- For extra potassium, make sure your diet includes plenty of fruits and beans.

- Milk and other dairy products can provide the calcium you need, although women often need extra calcium in supplemental form.

- To make sure you're ingesting enough magnesium, increase your intake of green leafy vegetables, nuts, seeds, and whole grains.

Check out the details on these easy steps in Chapters 9 and 10.

Planning realistic milestones to set the right pace

Modify your lifestyle one step at a time:

1. **Start by cutting back or eliminating smoking or chewing tobacco because this habit is by far the most dangerous.**

2. **Move on to reducing alcohol intake.**

3. **Go on to strengthen your heart and body through exercise after you've rid yourself of these habits (or have dramatically cut back on them).**

Pretend for a moment that your blood pressure is 140/85 mm Hg. You don't have any target-organ damage, but you have several risk factors including high cholesterol and a family history of heart disease. Lifestyle changes are in order. Your doctor warns you that you must quit your pack-a-day smoking habit, drop 20 pounds, and engage in 30 minutes of aerobic activity on a daily basis. You know you can't just turn your sedentary lifestyle around on a dime, so you chart out a plan like the one in Table 8-2 to incorporate your doctor's advice slowly but surely over a six-month time period.

Table 8-2	Sample Plan for Lifestyle Changes		
Time Period	*Daily Smoking Limit*	*Daily Exercise*	*Weight Loss*
Week 1	Half pack		
Week 2	5 cigarettes	Walk ½ mile	
Week 3	1 cigarette	Walk ¾ mile	
Week 4	None	Walk 1 mile	

Time Period	Daily Smoking Limit	Daily Exercise	Weight Loss
Weeks 5 to 8	None	Walk ½ mile & jog ½ mile	5 lb.
Weeks 9 to 12	None	Walk ¼ mile & jog ¾ mile	4 lb.
Weeks 13 to 16	None	Jog 1 mile	4 lb.
Weeks 17 to 20	None	Jog 1 mile	4 lb.
Weeks 21 to 24	None	Jog 1 mile	3 lb.

Plan and then chart your progress. You may also want to keep a daily diary of how many cigarettes you actually smoke, what you eat, and how much you exercise.

Tracking success and its spiraling effects

To keep a health record, go to www.lifeclinic.com and click on My Health Record. You can track your blood pressure, pulse, weight, cholesterol, blood sugar, personal health records, family health records, and a health checklist. The site also has extensive information on every aspect of high blood pressure, diabetes mellitus, cholesterol, and nutrition.

As you work on each change, notice how each new healthy habit affects many of the others. For example, increasing your level of exercise invigorates you and increases your tolerance for stress; as a result, you're less likely to smoke or drink alcohol when you want to relax. Similarly, the fewer cigarettes you smoke, the more your lung capacity increases and the easier exercising becomes *without* having to stop and catch your breath. These changes can help you to lose weight as well. *Note:* You may gain a few pounds as you stop smoking, but the benefits of stopping far outweigh (pun intended) those few pounds. Reducing the fat in your diet helps almost all the other risk factors as well. By the time you've gone through the list of lifestyle modifications, you'll feel like a new person.

Using laughter to lower blood pressure

You rarely find any mention of humor in a book about high blood pressure. This is probably because humor's place in the management of high blood pressure is so difficult to quantify, and scientists like to study only what they can measure. The effects of humor aren't in that category. I suppose you can take two groups of people, subject one to humorous experiences and the other to nonhumorous experiences, measuring their blood pressure before and after the experiences. That experiment may tell you about the immediate consequences of humor but not its long-term effects.

Understanding how laughter is good for what ails you

People such as author Norman Cousins and Joel Goodman, the head of the Humor Project, Inc. (see more on the Internet: www.humorproject.com), advocate humor for the management of most diseases. And high blood pressure, often associated with stress, seems like a natural focus for the positive effects of humor. The psychological and physiological effects of laughter have been demonstrated in a variety of settings — like teaching situations and the corporate environment. And mirth and merriment certainly reduce *stress hormone production* — the hormones known to raise blood pressure.

An interesting study in the *International Journal of Cardiology* (August 2001) indicated an inverse relationship between the tendency to find circumstances funny and the occurrence of coronary heart disease. A survey of 300 people assessed their tendency to laugh under a variety of situations in everyday life. The people with coronary heart disease were generally not laughers. Most of those without the disease were laughers. The results suggest that a tendency to laugh protects the heart.

Adding humor to your life

The last 30 years of experience with my patients convinces me that those who experience life with a certain degree of lightness, who are unwilling to take life too seriously, do much better than those who take it too seriously. I carry a card around from Dr. Joel Goodman that says, "Someday we will laugh about this. Why wait?" For most situations, it's an excellent prescription. Laughter signifies positive vibes to people. It adds to feelings of closeness, friendliness, and togetherness.

Even without definite proof of the value of humor, I recommend it as an important part of your high blood pressure treatment. How can you go about doing this? Find out for yourself what makes you laugh. Each person has a different source of amusement. Some people like clowns; others like standup comedians. Some prefer comedians like Eddie Murphy, and others think Woody Allen is a scream.

Here are a couple of ideas for bringing more laughter into your life:

✔ Find a reference book at your local library that lists movies by categories (humor, mystery, tragedy, and so forth). Pick out a few of the top-rated comedies. You may start with *Some Like It Hot, Annie Hall, Babe, Beverly Hills Cop,* or *Blazing Saddles. Seven Brides for Seven Brothers* and *Singin' in the Rain* may not make you laugh out loud (then again, they may), but you'll come away feeling much better about life in general.

> The old Marx Brothers and Bob Hope comedies or the newer stuff like the movies of Jack Black and Will Ferrell may appeal to you. Watch one of these at least once a week without fail. (No need to call me in the morning though!)
>
> ✔ Find a comedian you like and listen to his or her monologues in your car. Just be careful as you drive!

My bet is that this treatment helps bring your blood pressure down. Maybe lower blood pressure is a direct effect, or maybe humor just puts you into a good mood — a mood that helps you take your medications consistently, stay on your diet, and do your exercises. Either way, it's easy to swallow and contains no harmful side effects!

Like the other recommendations in this chapter, turning yourself on to humor is a lifestyle change for most people. So what if it's not backed up by the latest scientific evidence? You can't find a more pleasurable lifestyle change. I remember a quote from W. H. Auden in his book, *The Dyer's Hand and Other Essays* (Faber): "Among those whom I like or admire, I can find no common denominator. But among those whom I love, I can. All of them make me laugh."

He or she who laughs lasts.

Chapter 9

Choosing Foods that Lower High Blood Pressure

You are what you eat, the old saying goes. But it's truer than ever with high blood pressure. Weight loss, a well-balanced diet, and salt intake reduction can lower blood pressure. These approaches, however, haven't successfully kept blood pressure down in most patients. A new approach is needed.

In this chapter, you discover a new approach to healthy eating. I explain how it developed and proved effective, and I show you how to use it to reduce your blood pressure, no matter what your level is now. For people who want to reduce weight for whatever reason, I also provide a sensible, balanced program to help you get there. I try not to use the *D* (diet) word, but I do encourage you to follow a sensible nutritional program.

DASHing Down Your Blood Pressure

Based on study results at four major medical centers in the United States, the "Dietary Approach to Stop Hypertension" (DASH) diet was published in the *New England Journal of Medicine* (April 1997). All patients on the DASH diet successfully reduced their systolic and diastolic blood pressure (see Chapter 2 for more about these terms). Table 9-1 shows the average reduction in millimeters of mercury for the systolic blood pressure (SBP) and the diastolic blood pressure (DBP) for the various groups that followed the DASH diet.

Table 9-1	Average Reduction in Systolic (SBP) and Diastolic (DBP) Blood Pressure on the DASH Diet in Millimeters of Mercury	
Group	SBP	DBP
African Americans	6.9	3.7
Caucasians	3.3	2.4
Established high BP	11.6	5.3
No high BP	3.5	2.2

They achieved this reduction without special foods, food supplements, drugs, or weekly meetings. Furthermore, they achieved it without emphasizing weight loss by reducing kilocalories, without insisting on salt reduction, and without demanding exercise.

Are you intrigued? In the following sections, I describe the creation of the DASH diet and show you how to get started.

Leading up to DASH

DASH was created when doctors noted that vegetarians generally have lower blood pressure and a lower incidence of coronary heart disease (see Chapter 5) and brain attacks (see Chapter 7) than nonvegetarians. The reason isn't exactly clear. However, the big difference between vegetarians and nonvegetarians is that the former eat more fruits and vegetables than the latter. They also, of course, eat no meat and generally have less cholesterol and saturated fat in their pattern of eating.

Because a vegetarian program isn't a practical recommendation for the American public, scientists attempted to replicate the vegetarian program while permitting some meat. They looked for the substances in the food that could explain the fall in blood pressure.

The scientists recognized that a nutritional program with more fruits and vegetables has more potassium, which definitely affects blood pressure. The higher the potassium, the lower the blood pressure. So the increased potassium may be a partial explanation for the lower blood pressure, but it's not the entire story because similar amounts of potassium don't lower the blood pressure to the same extent unless salt is also reduced.

Note: The other important nutrients in vegetables and fruits are calcium and magnesium. However, studies haven't shown that these minerals lower blood pressure. And although fat intake reduction and the increase in fiber may lower blood pressure, researchers haven't determined their role in blood pressure control either.

The people who designed DASH decided that the mix of different nutrients may be responsible for the blood-pressure-lowering effect. To test their theory, they tried the combination on a large group of people, with an emphasis on African Americans, who have the highest rate of high blood pressure in the United States (as I note in Chapter 3).

Proving the value of DASH

The study involved 459 people with a systolic blood pressure under 160 mm Hg and a diastolic blood pressure of 80 to 95 mm Hg. In addition, the participants

- Were all older than 22
- Took no medications for high blood pressure
- Had to stop taking all vitamins and food supplements
- Couldn't drink more than 14 drinks of wine or other spirits per week
- Couldn't have poorly controlled diabetes, high blood fats, or a body mass index greater than 35 (see Table 9-5)

At the beginning of the study,

- Two out of three participants were African Americans.
- The mean age was 44 years.
- The average blood pressure of the group was 132/85 mm Hg with 29 percent having mild high blood pressure.
- Participants were mildly overweight with an average body mass index of 27.
- Twenty-seven percent were smokers.

For three weeks, the participants closely followed a common American diet (high in fats and total calories); then they were randomly broken into three groups:

- One group continued the usual American diet.
- The second group received a diet rich in fruits and vegetables.
- The third group was given DASH.

In addition, participants were given sufficient food so that they didn't lose weight, and they didn't have a decrease in salt intake. The diets continued for eight weeks.

After only two weeks, the usual diet group showed no change in blood pressure while the fruits-and-vegetables group reduced their blood pressures. But the DASH group had the greatest reduction in blood pressure, and they sustained this reduction for the entire study.

The average reduction in the DASH group's blood pressure was 6/3 mm Hg, but the best results were among the people with the highest blood pressures — 11/6 mm Hg.

Since the DASH study, other studies have accomplished the same excellent results using DASH, whether in an academic setting or in a primary-care outpatient practice. Some of these studies have shown other beneficial effects of DASH. For example:

- ✔ DASH lowered total blood cholesterol and low-density lipoprotein (LDL or *bad*) cholesterol.
- ✔ Blood levels of *homocysteine,* a substance associated with higher levels of coronary heart disease, were lowered.

Because most high blood pressure patients have mild stage 1 high blood pressure (140 to 159 mm Hg for systolic blood pressure or 90 to 99 mm Hg for diastolic blood pressure, whichever is higher) and most illnesses and deaths occur in that group, the extent of DASH's effects can have a significant impact on the health of Americans, especially those most at risk from high blood pressure.

DASH-Sodium, a second study that used various levels of sodium with the DASH program, showed that the lowest sodium level (1,500 mg daily) lowered blood pressure even more.

Getting with the program

The DASH program is usually based on a 2,000-kilocalorie-a-day diet. In the following sections, I provide you with the foods and servings in the program, sample menus, and tips for getting started and sticking with it.

If you find that following DASH is too difficult, don't hesitate to ask your doctor for a referral to a dietitian.

Specific foods and servings

The 2,000-kilocalorie DASH eating plan has the following foods and servings. If you need fewer kilocalories to maintain your weight, take the lower number of servings; if you need more kilocalories, take the higher number of servings. (See the later section "Reducing Your Weight to Lower Blood Pressure" for more information on determining the number of kilocalories you need.)

✔ **7 to 8 servings of grains and grain products daily**

A serving is 1 slice of bread, ½ bagel, ½ cup dry cereal, ½ cup cooked rice, pasta, or other cereal.

✔ **4 to 5 servings of vegetables daily**

A serving is 1 cup of raw, leafy vegetables, ½ cup cooked vegetables, 6 ounces vegetable juice.

✔ **4 to 5 servings of fruit daily**

A serving is 6 ounces of fruit juice, 1 medium fruit, ½ cup dried fruit, ½ cup of fresh, frozen, or canned fruit.

✔ **2 to 3 servings of low-fat or nonfat dairy products daily**

A serving is 1 cup 1-percent milk, 1 cup low-fat yogurt, and 1½ ounces nonfat cheese.

✔ **2 or fewer servings of meats, poultry, or fish daily**

A serving is 3 ounces of cooked lean meat, fish, or poultry.

✔ **2½ servings of fats daily**

A serving is 1 teaspoon oil, butter, margarine, mayonnaise, or 1 tablespoon regular or 2 tablespoons light salad dressing.

✔ **4 to 5 servings of nuts, seeds, or legumes per week**

A serving is ⅓ cup nuts, 2 tablespoons seeds, ½ cup cooked legumes, or 3 ounces tofu.

✔ **5 servings of sweets per week including 1 tablespoon sugar, 1 tablespoon jelly or jam, ½ ounce jelly beans, or 8 ounces of lemonade.**

Examples of good food choices in each group include

✔ **Grains and grain products:** English muffins, high-fiber cereals, oatmeal, pita bread, and whole wheat breads

✔ **Vegetables:** Artichokes, broccoli, carrots, collards, green beans, kale, peas, potatoes, spinach, squash, sweet potatoes, tomatoes, and turnip greens

✔ **Fruits:** Apples, apricots, bananas, dates, grapes, oranges, orange juice, grapefruit, grapefruit juice, mangos, melons, peaches, pineapples, prunes, raisins, strawberries, and tangerines

✔ **Dairy products:** Buttermilk — skim or low-fat; cheese — nonfat and part-skim mozzarella; milk — skim or 1-percent; yogurt — nonfat or low-fat

✔ **Fish, meats, and poultry:** Lean meats, poultry without skin, and no frying or sautéing

✔ **Nuts, seeds, and legumes:** Almonds, mixed nuts, peanuts, peanut butter, and walnuts; sesame or sunflower seeds; garbanzo beans, kidney beans, navy beans, pinto beans, lentils, split peas, and tofu

Sample menus

To make up your daily nutrition, Table 9-2 shows a sample menu.

Table 9-2		2,000 Kilocalorie DASH Menu	
Breakfast	**Lunch**	**Dinner**	**Snack**
3 grains	1 meat	1 meat	1 fruit
1 dairy	1 dairy	3 grains	1 grain
2 fruits	1 grain	3 vegetables	1 nuts
	1 fat		
1 fat	1 vegetable	1½ fat servings	
	1 fruit	1 fruit	

Eat a snack once daily.

Fill your own menu out following Table 9-3, or plan an entirely different day of meals, as Table 9-4 shows.

Table 9-3	Example of a 2,000 Kilocalorie DASH Meal Plan		
Breakfast	**Lunch**	**Dinner**	**Snack**
1 cup corn flakes	2 oz chicken	3 oz salmon	1 medium apple
1 cup 1% milk	½ oz low-fat cheddar	1 cup rice	1 slice wheat bread
1 banana	1 pita bread	1 cup squash	⅓ cup pecans
1 slice wheat toast	1 tsp margarine	1 cup spinach	
1 tbsp jam	1 cup raw carrots	1 tbsp light Italian dressing	
6 oz apple juice	1 orange	1½ oz low-fat Jack cheese	
1 tsp margarine			

Table 9-4   Another Example of a 2,000 Kilocalorie DASH Meal Plan

Breakfast	Lunch	Dinner	Snack
1 cup prune juice	2 oz lean beef	3 oz trout	1 orange
1 cup oatmeal	1 tsp BBQ sauce	1 cup brown rice	1 oz dried fruit
1 slice whole wheat	1 roll	1 cup three-bean salad	2 tbsp sunflower seeds
1 tsp margarine	1 cup boiled potatoes	1 tbsp low-fat dressing	
1 cup 1% milk	low-fat cheddar	1½ oz corn muffin	
1 banana	1 cup lettuce salad	1 tsp margarine	
	1 tbsp low-fat dressing	1 cup spinach	
	1 cup cranberry juice		

Helpful hints and resources

These suggestions can make the diet easier:

- ✔ Don't try to change all at once. Gradually reduce your meats and increase your fruits and vegetables.

- ✔ Increase fruit and vegetable servings by having two at each meal and two for a snack.

- ✔ If you're lactose intolerant, take lactase pills with the dairy foods or buy lactose-free milk.

- ✔ Use the *percent Daily Values* on food labels to pick the foods that are lowest in saturated fats, total fats, cholesterol, and salt.

- ✔ Reduce your fats so you're eating half your normal intake; emphasize vegetable fats over animal fats.

- ✔ Avoid soda, alcohol, and other sugar-sweetened drinks.

- ✔ Use fruits as desserts.

- ✔ Instead of meat, fish, or poultry, make grains (like pasta and rice), beans, and vegetables the center of the meal.

The government has a booklet about the DASH diet at www.nhlbi.nih. gov/health/public/heart/hbp/dash/. Other valuable sources of information about DASH include the following:

- DASH Diet Eating Plan at dashdiet.org/

- DASH, A Diet for All Diseases at www.cspinet.org/nah/dash.htm

- DASH Diet for Health at www.dashforhealth.com/

- DASH Diet Recipes at www.mayoclinic.com/health/dash-diet-recipes/RE00089

Recent reports from Harvard Medical School (*Journal of the American Medical Association*, November 2005) suggest that — in place of the carbohydrates like grains, cereals, and breads in the DASH diet — you can substitute protein (half from vegetable sources like beans, nuts, peas, seeds, and soy products) *or* monounsaturated fats (like grape seed oil, olive oil, avocado, almonds, cashews, hazelnuts, pumpkin seeds, and sesame seeds). The result is a further lowering of blood pressure and a positive effect on the fats in the blood (cholesterol), thereby reducing risk of a heart attack.

To find specific substitutions, go to www.omniheart.org/OmniDiets.pdf. You can alter your diet to include the food you prefer and still lower your blood pressure.

Reducing salt as you DASH

Chapter 10 tells you all about salt and high blood pressure. The bottom line is this: The less salt in your diet, the lower your blood pressure. If you want to combine DASH with low salt, here are some suggestions:

- Buy products that have *reduced sodium* or *no salt added* on their labels.

- Use herbs, spices, a little wine, lemon, lime, or vinegar instead of salt to flavor your food.

- Leave the saltshaker in the kitchen, away from the table, to help you fight the urge to add more salt when eating.

- Eat more unprocessed foods — Mother Nature knows what she's doing!

- Avoid high-salt condiments like soy sauce, teriyaki sauce, and monosodium glutamate (MSG).

- Reduce your intake of foods in brine and mustard, salt-cured foods, horseradish, ketchup, and Worcestershire sauce.

- Eat fruit and vegetable snacks instead of salty snack foods.

- Avoid salty foods when eating out.

Reducing Your Weight to Lower Blood Pressure

The fatter you are, the higher your blood pressure. More than 50 percent of the population is now overweight or obese as defined by the body mass index (BMI) shown in Table 9-5. In the following sections, you can calculate your BMI and find out whether your weight falls within the acceptable weight range for your height. You can also calculate the number of kilocalories you need to lose or maintain weight. If you do need to lose weight, I show you how to modify your diet to meet your new caloric needs.

For every 2.2 pounds of weight loss, your blood pressure drops by 1 mm of mercury systolic and 1 mm of mercury diastolic. In other words, if your blood pressure has been 135/85 and you lose 11 pounds, your blood pressure will fall to 130/80.

Calculating your ideal weight

In order to use weight loss to lower your blood pressure, you need to know your ideal weight. If you're already within the correct range of weights for your height, further weight loss will probably not lower your blood pressure much more. However, if you're overweight or obese, weight loss to your ideal range will significantly lower your blood pressure.

Based on studies of many healthy men and women, you can determine your ideal weight range in the following manner:

- ✔ If you're a woman, give yourself 100 pounds for being 5 feet tall and add 5 pounds for every inch over 5 feet.

    Example: If you're 5 feet 3 inches, your appropriate weight is 115 pounds. The ideal range is that weight plus or minus 10 percent, or 104 to 126 pounds.

- ✔ If you're a man, give yourself 106 pounds for being 5 feet tall and add 6 pounds for every inch over 5 feet.

    Example: A 5-foot-6-inch male should weigh about 142 pounds. The ideal weight range is then 128 to 156 pounds.

You can also use your BMI to determine whether you're under- or overweight. The BMI takes into account your height to determine whether your weight is too high. This is only fair. A 5-foot-4-inch woman who weighs 150 pounds is overweight, but a 5-foot-9-inch woman who weighs the same isn't overweight.

If you're good at math (or good with a calculator), you can determine your own BMI. (In case you forget to carry the *1*, I've done the work for you in Table 9-5.) Multiply your weight in pounds by 703. Divide the result by your height in inches. Divide that result by your height in inches again. This is your BMI in meters per kilogram squared. (You transfer pounds and inches into kilograms and meters with the 703 fudge factor.)

By definition, a BMI of 25 to 29.9 is overweight and a BMI of 30 or greater is obese. A BMI of 22 to 25 is normal.

> **Example:** A 150-pound, 5-foot-4-inch (64-inch) woman is overweight with a BMI of 27.5. A 150-pound, 5-foot-9-inch (69-inch) woman has a normal BMI of 22.2.

If you prefer the easy way of determining your BMI, use Table 9-5. Find your height in inches or meters in the left-hand column and move along that row until you reach your weight. Your BMI is at the top of that column.

Table 9-5						Body Mass Index Chart								
Body Mass Index (kg/ms²)														
	19	20	21	22	23	24	25	26	27	28	29	30	35	40
Height (inches/meters)	**Body Weight (pounds)**													
58/1.47	91	96	100	105	110	115	119	124	129	134	138	143	167	191
59/1.50	94	99	104	109	114	119	124	128	133	138	143	148	173	198
60/1.52	97	102	107	112	118	123	128	133	138	143	148	153	179	204
61/1.55	100	106	111	116	122	127	132	137	143	148	153	158	185	211
62/1.57	104	109	115	120	126	131	136	142	147	153	158	164	191	218
63/1.60	107	113	118	124	130	135	141	146	152	158	163	169	197	225
64/1.63	110	116	122	128	134	140	145	151	157	163	169	174	204	232
65/1.65	114	120	126	132	138	144	150	156	162	168	174	180	210	240
66/1.68	118	124	130	136	142	148	155	161	167	173	179	186	216	247
67/1.70	121	127	134	140	146	153	159	166	172	178	185	191	223	255
68/1.73	125	131	138	144	151	158	164	171	177	184	190	197	230	262
69/1.75	128	135	142	149	155	162	169	176	182	189	196	203	236	270
70/1.78	132	139	146	153	160	167	174	181	188	195	202	207	243	278

Body Mass Index (kg/ms²)													
19	20	21	22	23	24	25	26	27	28	29	30	35	40
Height (inches/ meters) Body Weight (pounds)													
71/1.80 136	143	150	157	165	172	179	186	193	200	208	215	250	286
72/1.83 140	147	154	162	169	177	184	191	199	206	213	221	258	294
73/1.85 144	151	159	166	174	182	189	197	204	212	219	227	265	302
74/1.88 148	155	163	171	179	186	194	202	210	218	225	233	272	311
75/1.90 152	160	168	176	184	192	200	208	216	224	232	240	279	319
76/1.93 156	164	172	180	189	197	205	213	221	230	238	246	287	328

Determining your daily caloric needs

Caloric needs are different depending on age, sex, and level of activity. For example, if a woman is pregnant or breast-feeding, she obviously needs more kilocalories. But if a person is trying to lose weight, then he needs to reduce the total kilocalories per day. When you know the appropriate weight for your height, you can determine the number of daily kilocalories to either maintain or reduce your present weight. Consider working with a dietitian to make sure you're getting the right nutrients while staying within your daily caloric limits.

A pound of fat contains 3,500 kilocalories. To lose a pound of fat, therefore, you must eat 3,500 kilocalories less than you need. You can do this a couple of ways:

- By reducing your daily intake 500 kilocalories for seven days
- By doing 200 kilocalories of exercise a day (see Chapter 12 for more about exercise) and reducing the diet by only 300 kilocalories daily.

For most people, a combination of diet and exercise seems to work much better than diet alone.

You don't have to lose weight all the way down to your appropriate range to benefit from weight loss. A loss of 5 to 10 percent of your current weight brings important benefits in terms of blood pressure, blood fats, and blood glucose (if diabetes is present).

Example: A 5-foot-3-inch woman who weighs 150 pounds should weigh within a range of 104 to 126 pounds, with 115 being her appropriate weight. At 115 pounds, she would require 115×10 or 1,150 kilocalories each day plus more, depending on her level of exercise. This calculation is derived from the heights and weights of a population of normal healthy men and women.

If she's sedentary, she's entitled to 10 percent more kilocalories, a total of 1,265 kilocalories daily. If she's moderately active, she gets 20 percent more, a total of 1,380 kilocalories daily. A very active woman may need 40 percent or more extra kilocalories to cover her exercise needs, up to 1,610 kilocalories daily.

By keeping her daily intake to 1,400 while doing 300 kilocalories of exercise daily, she can lose a pound of fat a week.

Adjusting your DASH diet

When you know your daily kilocaloric goal, you can go back to the DASH program and subtract or add servings appropriately. To figure out the DASH program at a lower caloric range without the assistance of a dietitian, Table 9-6 shows the breakdown of servings for 2,000-, 1,800-, and 1,500-kilocalorie DASH programs.

Table 9-6	Daily Servings Comparison for 2,000, 1,800, and 1,500 kilocalorie DASH		
Food Group	*2,000 Kilocalorie*	*1,800 Kilocalorie*	*1,500-Kilocalorie Servings*
Grains	8	8	5½
Vegetables	4	4	4
Fruits	5	4	4
Dairy foods	3	3	3
Meats and fish	2	1¾	1¾
Fats and oils	2½	2½	1½
Nuts and seeds	1	1	¾
Sweets	5 per week		

Without a doubt, the simplest way to lose weight successfully — *without* eating foods you don't like — is the half-portion plan. Many of my patients (including those who come from a variety of ethnic backgrounds with different food preferences) have been able to lose weight and keep it off using this method. When they eat at home, they cut the portion in half and save the other half for another meal. When they eat out, they share an entrée with their partner. Most restaurants give you much more food than you should eat at one meal. Take advantage of it!

If you're following the DASH diet, you can significantly reduce calories with some simple substitutions:

- ✔ Use fat-free or low-fat condiments
- ✔ Reduce the oil or dressing in half
- ✔ Drink low-fat milk
- ✔ Check labels for added sugar
- ✔ Avoid fruits canned in sugary syrup
- ✔ Add fruit to plain yogurt
- ✔ Snack on carrot sticks, celery sticks, plain popcorn, or rice cakes
- ✔ Avoid caloric drinks; stick to water with lemon or lime

Ghrelin: The reason you may have trouble losing weight

Many of my patients have wondered why losing weight seems to get harder the more weight you lose. Interestingly, a good scientific reason lies in *ghrelin* (the Hindu word for *growth*), a recently discovered hormone that stimulates growth-hormone secretion from the brain. This hormone is also called the *hunger* hormone because it travels through the blood from the upper part of the stomach to the brain, where it stimulates the appetite. Scientists have discovered that a person's ghrelin normally rises just before meals and falls when food is taken. But if a person loses weight by dieting, the levels of ghrelin before meals are much higher, causing greater hunger.

A person who undergoes stomach bypass surgery (the upper part of the stomach is excluded from the digestive tract) has little ghrelin. This reduction of the hunger hormone helps to explain the loss of appetite after that surgery.

Trying Other Diets

Sometimes you need a boost to get you going in the right direction towards weight loss and the resulting reduction in blood pressure. I don't insist that my patients follow a balanced nutrition plan all the time as long as I'm certain that they're generally getting the good nutrition they need. You may need a special plan to get you started, and then you can continue on a healthy, balanced program like DASH. For example, one of my patients eats nothing but rice and water one week a month and then eats balanced meals the rest of the time. He has lost a significant amount of weight, has come off all blood pressure medication, and has a blood pressure anyone would envy. He looks and feels great.

Weight loss is difficult for many reasons. In my experience, most patients do well initially but tend to return to old habits. Still, losing weight and keeping it off is definitely possible. At one time, only 1 out of 20 people who lost weight kept it off. Now the figure is closer to one in five. You should certainly check with a dietitian or your physician for new ideas about weight loss.

How do successful losers do it?

What's different about the people who have lost weight and kept it off? The National Weight Loss Registry surveyed more than 3,000 people to find out. The registry surveyed people who had lost at least 30 pounds and kept it off for at least one year.

The people had a starting BMI of 36, lost an average of 71 pounds, and currently had an average BMI of 25. Here are some of their characteristics:

- 74 percent had one or both overweight parents.

- 20 percent were overweight by age 18.

- They had recycled (gained and lost) an average of 271 pounds over their lifetime.

- Most had lost weight in the usual ways: restricting foods, portion control, counting kilocalories, and limiting fats.

- Their average kilocalorie intake was 1,300 kilocalories per day for women and 1,650 for men to maintain weight loss.

- Their average weekly kilocalorie expenditure from exercise was 2,800 kilocalories.

- 55 percent used a program such as Weight Watchers, Overeaters Anonymous, or a dietitian; 45 percent lost weight on their own.

- 77 percent reported a medical or emotional trigger that caused them to lose weight successfully.

If you study these characteristics, you find that these people aren't following strange plans to lose weight. They're using ordinary nutritional plans that are usually balanced, in addition to exercise and sometimes outside help.

Successfully losing weight and maintaining it also requires a willingness to exercise. Chapter 12 is all about exercise both for health and for weight loss. If, for some reason, you can't move your legs to exercise, you can get a satisfactory workout using your upper body. Most people who are successful at weight loss maintenance describe exercise as a key part of their success.

The following diets aren't balanced diets and shouldn't be your nutritional plan for more than several weeks to get you going. Unfortunately, they're generally associated with *regaining* the weight if they become your primary program because they're usually boring, repetitious, and have little to do with the pleasure of eating.

- ✔ **Very-low-kilocalorie diets:** These diets provide 400 to 800 kilocalories a day of protein and carbohydrate with supplemental vitamins and minerals. They're safe when supervised by a physician and when you need rapid weight loss (like in the case of a heart condition). They result in rapid initial weight loss and less need for high blood pressure medication. In fact, if you continue your medication, you may suffer dizziness.

- ✔ **Animal-protein diets** (such as the Atkins diet): Food is limited to animal protein, vitamins, and minerals in an effort to maintain body protein. Patients often complain of hair loss, and they rapidly regain weight when they discontinue the diet. This is not a balanced diet.

- ✔ **Fasts:** A fast means giving up all food for a period of time and taking only water, vitamins, and minerals. A fast is such a drastic change from normal eating habits that most patients don't remain on it for very long. As a result, they regain the weight.

Using Outside Help

The dietitian can be a tremendous source of information on all aspects of nutrition. He can help you determine your correct weight and the ideal number of kilocalories per day to reach that weight. Your physician or local hospital can provide the name of a reputable dietitian.

Other programs have also proved to be valuable for some people. Many of these programs provide all the food you care to eat, making it exceedingly easy to follow them (although they can also be exceedingly expensive). These programs emphasize gradual weight loss and a connection to more normal eating habits, both of which seem to be a more successful way to lose weight.

- **Jenny Craig:** This organization provides the food that you eat, which you must pay for. It offers information on food behavior modification.

- **Weight Watchers:** This organization emphasizes slow weight loss, exercise, and behavior modification. It charges for weekly attendance at its meetings, which you can find all over the world. Although it doesn't require you to purchase any products, its brand of food is available for purchase. Weight Watchers has developed a point program that allows you to eat what you want — as long as the total is within your point allowance each day. After you reach your goal, you can belong to the organization for free as long as you stay at that weight or near it. Weight Watchers is very motivating.

Chapter 10

Keeping Salt Out of Your Diet

• •

• •

Since the previous edition of this book, many laboratories have studied the effect of salt on the blood pressure and the kidneys. None of the newly published information causes me to change the basic information in this chapter. Although salt is not to blame for high blood pressure, reduction in salt intake can reduce the blood pressure in most cases. In addition, according to an article in the June 2006 *American Journal of Nephrology*: "There is consistent experimental evidence to link increased salt exposure with kidney tissue damage."

The Salt Institute, a nonprofit association of salt producers founded in 1914, would have you believe that eating salt doesn't raise your blood pressure *and* that there's no proof that higher blood pressure is harmful to your health. Don't believe them! With rare exceptions, every expert in the field of high blood pressure recommends reducing salt consumption to lower high blood pressure.

The United States is by far the world's largest producer of salt. We make about 46.5 million metric tons annually compared with the next country, China, which makes 37.1-million metric tons, followed by Germany at 16 million, India at 15 million, Canada at 14.1 million, and Australia at 11.2 million. These six countries account for 140 million of the 209-million metric tons produced each year in the world. Although only 6 percent of that salt is for human consumption, these same countries tend to consume the most per person — a situation that helps explain their equally high prevalence of high blood pressure.

In this chapter, I explain how your salt intake can elevate your blood pressure, and I show how research has provided overwhelming evidence to this effect. Also, you discover how sensitivity to salt can increase your blood pressure, how you can decrease the amount of salt in your food, what foods are low or high in salt, and what's in a low-salt diet. You *can* eat without salting down your plate. I hope that by the end of the chapter you can put your saltshaker away, never to be seen again — or at least reduce your salt intake so it does you no harm.

Making the Connection between Salt and High Blood Pressure

Salt, which contains 40 percent sodium and 60 percent chloride, is critical to your life. You can't live without it. Sodium helps maintain your blood's water content, balances the acids and bases in your blood, and is necessary for the electrical charges in your nerves that move your muscles.

Researchers generally believe that a kidney's inability to excrete salt is responsible for salt-induced high blood pressure. To compensate for this inability, the body increases blood pressure so the kidney can filter more salt, which then enters the urine. This increased blood pressure helps eliminate more salt, but it also puts a strain on the body's arteries and sets the downward spiral of blood-pressure damage in motion — a vicious cycle.

Food labels list the amount of sodium, not salt, in the food. The Dietary Guidelines for Americans from the United States Department of Health and Human Services, as well as from the American Heart Association, recommend 2,400 milligrams (mg) daily for adults or 1 teaspoon of salt (2,300 mg to be exact). The average American consumes 5,000 mg of sodium daily — twice the necessary amount. *Note:* Normal sodium balance can be maintained with 500 mg daily (a little more than ¼ teaspoon of salt), so Americans are eating ten times as much as they really need!

Canada, Australia, the United Kingdom, and Portugal all have about the same recommendation of 2,400 mg of salt. Some countries — Germany (4,000 mg), the Netherlands (3,600 mg), and Belgium (3,500 mg) — are more liberal, and at least one country, Sweden (800 mg), is more restrictive than the United States.

"Where is all this salt coming from?" you may ask. Two sources primarily:

- ✔ Many foods are a natural source of salt (like meat and fish).
- ✔ Many foods contain salt added during processing (prepared soup and crackers, for example).

For more information on the amount of salt in the foods you eat, see the "Lowering Your Salt Intake" section later in this chapter.

Proving the Salt-Blood Pressure Connection

An experiment that involved the overabundant consumption of salt would be hard to do on human beings because their salt intake is so high to begin with. Also, a person would need to take an unpalatable amount of additional salt to significantly raise his body's salt level. However, studies of people with high blood pressure who undergo periods of salt reduction are easily performed.

Although reducing salt intake hasn't been proven to always lower blood pressure, studies have shown that eating less salt, in most cases, leads to lower blood pressure and fewer instances of heart attack and brain attack. For example, the blood pressure measurements of individuals with a great craving for salt were extremely high when they ate an abundance of salt. When the same individuals reduced their salt intake, blood pressures dropped significantly.

Examining early experiments

In the early twentieth-century, the first experiments on the salt-blood pressure connection showed that blood pressure fell as salt was reduced. You can find these studies in the *Archives of General Medicine* (February 1904).

A low-salt diet lowered blood pressure in half of the patients who had high blood pressure. In the rest of the patients, changes may have been irreversible (in other words, the blood pressure no longer responded to salt deprivation alone), or some patients may not have been salt sensitive (I discuss salt sensitivity later in this chapter).

In the *American Journal of Medicine* (March 1948), a study established without a doubt that salt restriction lowers blood pressure. Shortly afterwards, however, the first *diuretics* (blood pressure drugs that increase salt and water excretion; see Chapter 13) came on the market. As a result, salt restriction as a means of lowering blood pressure fell out of favor. However, as side effects from these drugs became a problem, salt restriction became more popular again.

In 1988, the Intersalt Study, a huge study of over 10,000 people from many nations, showed that salt intake is directly related to the rise of both systolic and diastolic blood pressures with age (see Chapter 2 for more about these types of blood pressure). The researchers concluded that reducing salt intake by 1 teaspoon daily from age 25 to 55 can reduce the blood pressure by 9 mm Hg. Many people with prehypertension can lower their blood pressure to normal just by restricting salt. ***Note:*** People who lived where the salt intake was lowest had no increase in blood pressure with age.

Taking some study results with a grain of salt

At first glance, the evidence for the connection between excess salt and high blood pressure appears overwhelming. However, a few studies seem to show that salt isn't dangerous to your health. In one particular study reported in *Hypertension* (June 1995), Alderman wrote that heart attacks increased among the men who had the lowest salt intake. ***Note:*** This study had a number of problems associated with it. The most serious problem was that the patients had their salt intake tested only one time in four years; their intake was considered high or low based on that single test. The average of multiple tests would have been more accurate.

Considering chloride's effects on blood pressure

Current professional opinion maintains that sodium alone doesn't raise blood pressure. Instead, the combination of sodium *and* chloride raises blood pressure. Studies at the University of California in San Francisco by Dr. R. Curtis Morris and his associates have shown that some people are sensitive to both sodium and chloride, but others are sensitive to chloride even when it's not combined with sodium.

In rats that are genetically prone to high blood pressure, potassium chloride (a common replacement for sodium chloride — salt) can raise blood pressure just as much as sodium chloride does. Whether this finding is applicable to human beings is uncertain at the present time. However, 15 years ago, Morris and his associates showed that sodium bicarbonate (baking soda) does not raise blood pressure in salt-sensitive people. As a result, they recommend that potassium bicarbonate or potassium citrate (*not* potassium chloride) replace sodium chloride.

A study of people with high blood pressure in Germany (October 1990 *Hypertension*) offers evidence that chloride plays a part in high blood pressure. A group of patients with high blood pressure was given either potassium chloride or potassium citrate in place of sodium chloride. Those who received potassium citrate lowered their blood pressure significantly, but those who received potassium chloride did not. ***Note:*** The potassium in fruits and vegetables is not potassium chloride. This difference may help to explain the positive effects of fruits and vegetables on high blood pressure (see Chapter 9 for more information).

Reviewing recent studies

A Finnish study in the September 2006 *Progress in Cardiovascular Disease* showed that a one-third decrease in salt intake over 30 years led to a drop in systolic pressure of more than 10 mm of mercury in both systolic and diastolic pressure throughout the population. In addition, the population showed a 75 percent decrease in deaths due to heart attacks and brain attacks. After reviewing this study, I threw out my saltshakers!

This is a truly remarkable accomplishment. The Finns believe they have been able to greatly reduce blood pressure and its complications — heart attacks and brain attacks — by the following methods:

- ✔ Hundreds of articles in leading newspapers since 1978 have emphasized the *toxicity* of salt.

- ✔ Extensive reports to the public have recommended sodium-reduced, potassium- and magnesium-enriched, healthier salt alternatives.

- ✔ Food manufacturers, the major source of salt in Finnish diets, have to add *High Salt Content* to the label if a product's percentage of salt is higher than the allowable amount. Rather than put this label on their foods, they have lowered the salt content. (They're also allowed to label their food *Low Salt Content* if the product meets certain levels.)

- ✔ Restaurants are allowed to label their food *Pansalt* if it has reduced sodium and increased potassium and magnesium salts. Owners find this to be a good marketing technique.

Salt through human history

Human beings who lived away from the seashores several thousand years ago didn't eat much salt because most salt comes from the sea. They existed on no more than 200 to 400 milligrams (less than ½ teaspoon) of salt each day because the human body generally conserves it. When an athlete sweats, he puts out sweat with less and less salt as exercise continues. Meanwhile, the kidneys return all the filtered salt back to the body.

When people discovered that salt preserved and extended the life of some foods (about 3,000 BC), salt became much more valuable. At the same time, the salty taste of food became the norm and unsalted food was considered bland. At that time salt became such a sought-after commodity that governments began to put a tax on salt transactions to gain revenue. The salt tax was a major reason for the French Revolution.

Around 1850, salt became cheap as methods of producing it improved. Salt consumption rose enormously. By the nineteenth century, people consumed as much as 20 grams (or 4 teaspoons) of salt daily. Luckily, with refrigeration, adding salt as a preservative to food began to decline.

Determining Whether You're Salt Sensitive

Salt was first shown to raise blood pressure in rats in experiments published in the February 1957 *Journal of the American Dietetic Association*. At the end of nine months, the rats that had consumed the most salt had the highest blood pressure. However, not all rats in this study showed this increase in blood pressure; some were sensitive to salt and some weren't. This study showed that the sensitivity was hereditary, that is, passed down through the genes.

Salt sensitivity in humans is similar:

✔ When children of parents with high blood pressure eat salt in large quantities, they can't get rid of it through their urine as rapidly as children of parents who don't have high blood pressure.

✔ When children of parents with high blood pressure eat salt, their blood pressure is higher if both parents have high blood pressure than if only one parent has high blood pressure.

✔ When children of parents without high blood pressure eat salt in large quantities, their blood pressure isn't elevated at all.

These findings are published in the *Journal of Hypertension* (April 1986).

About half the United States population (and, where studied, half the populations in other industrialized countries) is salt sensitive. This high percentage has caused plenty of confusion in experiments meant to show the effects of salt on human beings. Among the people who tend to be more salt sensitive are

✔ Elderly individuals (over age 65)

✔ Overweight individuals

✔ African Americans

✔ Diabetics

✔ People with kidney disease

Reduce your salt intake whether you're salt sensitive or not because

✔ If you are sensitive, the reduction helps to reduce your blood pressure.

✔ If you're not sensitive, the reduced salt intake can reduce the extra water that your body naturally retains due to salt.

Linking salt sensitivity and metabolic syndrome

Salt sensitivity seems to be the cause of high blood pressure in *metabolic syndrome,* a condition that includes high blood pressure, decreased sensitivity to the body's insulin, usually increased abdominal fat (due to overweight), high levels of the fat triglyceride and LDL (bad) cholesterol, and low levels of the good (HDL) cholesterol. This condition is present in more than 50 million Americans. With their salt restricted, many people with metabolic syndrome experience a significant fall in their blood pressure to normal levels.

Lowering Your Salt Intake

Surprisingly, you're responsible for only 15 percent of the salt in your diet, and food naturally has about 10 percent of your salt. This means the food industry is responsible for 75 percent of the salt you consume. For example, the following additives contain plenty of it:

- **Color Developer:** Promotes the development of color in meats and sauerkraut

- **Fermentation Controller:** Slows the process of fermentation in cheeses, sauerkraut, and baked goods

- **Binder:** Keeps meat together as it cooks

- **Texture Aid:** Allows dough to expand and not tear

For these and other reasons, salt is a part of food *processing* — it's not all for taste.

The only way to successfully reduce the salt in your diet is by switching from processed foods to fresh foods or by selecting low-salt processed foods.

Buying low-salt foods

The Food and Drug Administration has definite guidelines for food companies regarding a product's salt-content description. Keep these terms in mind and make a point of buying low-salt foods on your next trip to the grocery store:

- **Low sodium** means less than 140 mg sodium in a portion.

- **Very low sodium** means less than 35 mg sodium in a portion.

- **Sodium free** means less than 5 mg sodium in a portion.

- ✔ **Reduced sodium** food contains 25 percent less sodium than the original food item.

- ✔ **Light in sodium** food has 50 percent less sodium than the original food item.

- ✔ **Unsalted, No salt added,** or **Without added salt** means absolutely no salt has been added to a food that's normally processed with salt.

Take time to read the Nutrition Facts label on food items. Avoid items that contain more than 180 milligrams of sodium.

Avoiding high-salt foods

Table 10-1 shows the processed foods that are particularly high in salt. Avoid eating these foods as much as possible. Fortunately, after many years of urging and recommendations from health organizations, manufacturers have begun to lower the salt in foods, so you may find several of these items in a low-salt form. Check the food label.

Table 10-1	Prepared High-Salt Foods	
Anchovies	Condiments	Pickles
Bacon	Cooking sauces	Salad dressings
Bouillon cubes	Cottage cheese	Salsa
Canned soups	Croutons	Sausage
Canned tuna	Gravy	Sea salt
Canned vegetables	Ham	Soy sauce
Cheese	Hot dogs	Spaghetti sauce
Cold cuts	Olives	Tomato or vegetable juice

Going on a low-salt diet

Besides avoiding high-salt foods, you can make a few other changes to lower your salt intake:

✔ Cook with herbs, spices, fruit juices, and vinegars, instead of salt, to add flavor.

✔ Eat fresh vegetables.

✔ Keep the saltshaker in the kitchen cupboard instead of at the table, where it's so easy to use.

✔ Use less salt than the recipe calls for.

✔ Select low-salt canned foods or rinse your food with water.

✔ Select low-salt frozen dinners.

✔ Use high-salt condiments like ketchup and mustard sparingly.

✔ Snack on fresh fruits instead of salted crackers or chips.

✔ When eating out, ask that your food be prepared with only a little salt. Request your salad dressing *on the side* so you can control the amount.

Be careful of salt substitutes because some contain sodium. You may end up eating so much of the substitute to get that salty taste that your total sodium intake is just as high as using salt. Check the label! Some salt substitutes contain potassium and should not be used by people with impaired kidney function.

Combining a low-salt diet with DASH

Chapter 9 explains the DASH nutritional program in detail. Combine DASH with a low-salt diet to get the maximum blood-pressure-lowering effect. Some recommendations for the various food groups in DASH are as follows:

✔ **Grains:** Check the salt content of all prepared grain foods, and keep the sodium less than 180 mg in each serving. Avoid any salted grain foods such as salted popcorn.

✔ **Fruits:** Avoid dried fruits with salt.

✔ **Vegetables:** Eat fresh vegetables and read the label on prepared vegetables.

✔ **Meats:** Eat fresh meats, fish, and poultry; avoid salt-cured products.

✔ **Dairy products:** Read the label and avoid products with more than 180 mg of sodium per serving.

✔ **Fats:** Avoid high-salt salad dressings and salted butter.

✔ **Nuts and seeds:** Avoid salted varieties.

✔ **Sweets:** Check the box and stay away from prepared mixes that contain more than 180 mg of sodium per serving.

Chapter 11

Avoiding Tobacco, Alcohol, and Caffeine

*S*uppose I told you that even if you're older than 45 years of age, you can do all the following:

✔ Improve your work performance, your sex life, and, if you're pregnant, the health of you and your baby

✔ Increase your social activities and the possibility of living longer

✔ Reduce the possibility of getting a driving ticket, contracting a sexually-transmitted disease, and committing suicide or homicide

✔ Lower your blood pressure

Would you make a little sacrifice? Of course. All that you need to do is quit smoking (or chewing smokeless tobacco), drinking alcohol excessively, and drinking coffee. You're probably thinking those are easy for me to say but much harder for you to do. Lucky for you, I give you every available tool to make this lifestyle improvement as easy as possible. Nothing you do for your health can make a greater difference than cutting out tobacco and significantly reducing your consumption of alcohol and caffeine.

In this chapter, I take up each one of these dangerous habits individually and discuss how they affect your blood pressure. I also discuss how eliminating these poisons from your life can help lower your blood pressure and make your mind and body healthier in the process.

Tobacco, alcohol, and caffeine most often go together. The person who smokes more often than not is the person who drinks too much alcohol and caffeine. Tobacco, alcohol, and caffeine represent a triple threat to your health. But within that triple threat may also be triple salvation. Reducing or eliminating one of these poisons often leads to a reduction or elimination of one or both of the others. The tendency to have that cigarette with your scotch or your coffee is eliminated if you don't drink the scotch or the coffee.

Playing with Fire: Tobacco and High Blood Pressure

When you play with fire, you get burned. When you smoke, you run the risk of getting burned inside and out. Whether tobacco is smoked, chewed, or taken in by any other means, the *nicotine* (a colorless, poisonous chemical used to kill insects) in the tobacco raises the blood pressure. The more you smoke, the higher the nicotine level in your blood and the higher your blood pressure. To a large extent, this effect accounts for the great increase in brain attacks (see Chapter 7), heart attacks (see Chapter 5), and pain in the legs due to poor circulation in smokers, sometimes leading to amputation.

Nicotine raises your blood pressure by constricting your blood vessels. The oxygen in your blood decreases as the nicotine directly stimulates the production of *epinephrine* (also known as *adrenaline,* a hormone that raises blood pressure) in the adrenal gland. After tobacco use raises blood pressure, you're at risk for all the medical consequences of high blood pressure (Part II describes these), not to mention diseases such as mouth and lung cancer associated with smoking.

Numerous studies have shown that smoking and chewing tobacco raise blood pressure and that when you stop using tobacco products, your blood pressure falls. The latest such study in the *Journal of Hypertension* (March 2007) comes from China. For ten years, researchers followed 10,525 men and women who did not initially have high blood pressure. At the end of the study, key predictors of future high blood pressure included age, weight, excess alcohol, and cigarette smoking. Do you need more evidence than that?

The reason people have so much trouble giving up smoking is because they're nicotine dependent. But along with the nicotine, cigarette companies generously provide more than 60 chemicals that are known to cause cancer and more than 4,000 other chemicals in each cigarette.

Cigarettes (and smokeless tobacco like chewing tobacco) deserve their own book, but in the following sections, I give you enough evidence of the dangers of tobacco and enough helpful advice to quit that you'd have to be a real dummy not to stop immediately, if not sooner. Consider this: Drugs that cause only a small fraction of the illness and death that tobacco can be blamed for have been taken off the market. So why are cigarettes still sold legally and advertised in prestigious magazines? The answer to that question lies squarely at the feet of government and the millions of dollars in cigarette sales that are turned around and used to influence that government. Some day you'll look back on these times and ask yourself, "Could I really have been that stupid?"

You benefit from stopping smoking no matter your age or physical condition.

Examining the extent of the problem

Forty-six million Americans smoked in 2001. The problem is even greater in other countries. One-third of the population of the world older than age 15 smokes, a total of 1.4 billion people. In many other countries, more than half the adult population smokes.

The overall rate of smoking in America has declined from 25 percent in 1993 to 22.8 percent in 2001 according to the United States smoking statistics of the National Institutes of Health. The federal government has set a goal of 12 percent by 2010. However, this goal isn't achievable at the current rate. The decline in other countries has been even less.

Regarding the age of smokers, about 18 percent of youths age 12 to 17 years smoke, 27 percent of young adults age 18 to 25 years smoke, 22 percent of people age 26 to 44 years of age smoke, and only 10 percent of adults aged 65 and older continue to smoke. Most tobacco users begin before the age of 18 despite the tobacco companies' continued *efforts* to avoid attracting that age group.

At a rate of 33 percent, Native Americans lead among the various ethnic groups in percent of smokers. Caucasians and African Americans have the same rate of about 24 percent, and about 17 percent of Hispanics are smokers. Only 12 percent of Asians and Pacific Islanders are smokers.

People *can* stop smoking. The evidence is 46 million *former* smokers in the United States in 2002.

The direct costs of smoking (like health insurance costs, use of medical care, and expenses due to medical care) amount to more than 60 billion dollars per year in the United States alone. The indirect costs (like loss of work due to smoking-related illness and loss in productivity from deaths due to smoking) add another 90 billion or so dollars. Many experts suggest that cigarettes should have a much higher tax to meet part of these costs. This added cost would not only help to pay for the self-inflicted diseases of smokers but also discourage the purchase of cigarettes in the first place. The current gradual decline in smoking among the population is the result of the last increase in cigarette taxes.

Putting one foot in the grave

Blood pressure elevation is just one of smoking's many consequences. Other smoking-related complications are as follows:

- Lung cancer is 20 times more likely among smokers than nonsmokers.

- Cancers of the mouth and throat as well as the bladder are more likely among smokers. The connection isn't as clear, but smoking is also likely to increase the possibility of cancers of the liver, large intestine, pancreas, kidney, and cervix in women.

- Coronary heart disease is much more common among smokers, whether they have increased blood pressure or not.

- Brain attacks (see Chapter 7) are more common among smokers — again, regardless of elevated blood pressure.

- Bleeding from rupture of the large blood vessel in the abdomen is more common.

- Chronic lung disease is most often the result of smoking.

- Lung growth rate is reduced among adolescents who smoke.

- Women who smoke have trouble conceiving a baby, and if they do, they're more likely to miscarry. Women who smoke also tend to start menopause at a younger age.

- Smoking reduces bone density and increases the risk of fractures, especially in older women.

- Tobacco dries and wrinkles the skin while it yellows your teeth, fingers, and fingernails.

- A correlation exists between smoking and depression.

Do you need more reasons to stop smoking? Just keep this in mind: If you smoke, you're not utterly cool; you're an utter fool.

Combating secondhand smoke

Secondhand smoke (also called *environmental tobacco smoke* or *sidestream smoke*) is mostly inhaled from the burning end of someone else's cigarette. This smoke can be just as deadly as smoke from the other end (the *mainstream* smoke) and perhaps more so because it's mostly unfiltered and contains more of the poisons, including nicotine (check back to earlier in this section for more on this). Each year in the United States alone, secondhand smoke causes 3,000 nonsmoker deaths due to lung cancer and 55,000 nonsmoker deaths due to heart and blood vessel disease.

Don't become a victim of secondhand smoke. Just follow these guidelines:

- ✔ Allow no one to smoke in your home or car.
- ✔ Never smoke with children around.
- ✔ Improve ventilation if exposure to smoke can't be avoided.
- ✔ Insist that offices and bars be completely smoke-free.

Turning a cheek to smokeless tobacco

Smokeless tobacco is tobacco that you chew or put into your nostrils. Types of smokeless tobacco include

- ✔ Snuff, which people in the United States place between the cheek and the gum and which Europeans sniff into the nose
- ✔ Chewing tobacco, a wad of tobacco placed inside the cheek and chewed on to extract the juices

In the process of using either one, a great deal of saliva is produced, forcing the user to spit frequently. How handsome is that!

Smokeless tobacco provides at least twice as much nicotine as a cigarette. Eight to ten chews a day is equivalent to the nicotine content of 40 cigarettes! So, smokeless tobacco damages the heart and blood vessels over the long term, and it has greater and longer effects on blood pressure than cigarettes. In addition, smokeless tobacco is filled with agents that cause cancer.

Smokeless tobacco can't help you quit smoking. In fact, it

- ✔ Is just as addictive as cigarettes, if not more
- ✔ Can't get rid of your nicotine cravings
- ✔ Discolors your teeth and sours your breath
- ✔ Creates cancer in your throat, voice box, and esophagus

Not exactly great advertising material!

Giving up tobacco: All wins, no losses

Why should you give up something you find pleasurable and that may help you keep those extra pounds off? As far as the pounds, plan to get rid of those with more exercise and fewer kilocalories (head to Chapter 12 to find out more about exercise). As for the pleasure, the short- and long-term health consequences when you quit are as follows:

- ✔ The healing starts within 12 hours as the carbon monoxide levels in your body fall. Your heart and lungs begin to function more normally, lowering your blood pressure and heart rate.

- ✔ Your taste buds and your sense of smell return in a few days.

- ✔ Your face wrinkles far less as you age.

- ✔ If you're attempting to get pregnant, achieving pregnancy is easier; after you're pregnant, the pregnancy proceeds in a healthier manner.

- ✔ Your smoker's cough diminishes after a few days, though it may last for a while as your rejuvenated lungs begin to mobilize and expel the gunk accumulated over years of smoking.

- ✔ The stench of stale smoke and the mess of cigarette butts are gone, along with the expense of smoking and the time wasted buying cigarettes and finding a place to smoke.

- ✔ Your risk of early death is the same as a nonsmoker's after 10 to 15 years of no cigarettes, depending on how long you smoked before stopping.

- ✔ After five years, the risk of cancer of the mouth and throat — along with bladder cancer and cancer of the cervix in women — significantly diminishes.

- ✔ After ten years, you have half the chance of developing lung cancer than if you continued to smoke.

Obviously, the healthy consequences of quitting tobacco are reason enough for you to stop, but other reasons may sway you just as much:

- ✔ A loved one may tell you that the cigarettes go or you go. After all, kissing a smoker is like licking an ashtray.

- ✔ The money you save may provide a down payment for a new car, buy a new computer, or just allow you to keep eating. If you're a two-pack-a-day smoker, cigarettes at the cheapest price in 2007 cost you a minimum of $1,600 a year.

- ✔ You freeze while standing outside several times a day just to get your nicotine fix.

- ✔ You can use the time you save by *not* going to the store or standing outside to exercise or do some other healthy activity.

- ✔ You're getting as disgusted as I am with the cigarette butts that litter city streets.

- ✔ The days that you add onto your life aren't just a matter of time. They're productive, healthy days — days that you may have spent gasping for breath, with an oxygen tube in your nose, and too short of breath to walk over to your grandchild and hug her.

✔ Your children do as you do, not as you say. They probably won't smoke if you don't, which means your grandchildren won't either. So if *you* stop, you may prolong the lives and improve the quality of life of generations to come.

Kicking the habit

The last few years have seen a smoking-cessation-treatment revolution. Psychotherapy started it, and it was followed by nicotine gum and then nicotine patches. Today's drugs take away the craving for nicotine but don't contain it. In this section, you can find a method that appeals to you. I know you want to quit smoking because more than 70 percent of adults have expressed a desire to stop. Now's your chance!

No one way works for all people. Try each one. If it doesn't work for you, try another technique. Something will click eventually.

Keys to quitting

You must take five steps to ensure that you quit and don't relapse. If you do relapse, start with these same five steps next time:

1. **Prepare yourself.**

   Set a quit date and make it special. After all, your body is being reborn. Your birth date will do nicely — a day of celebration for the rest of your life.

   In addition:

   • Make a list of reasons to quit.

   • Improve your fitness, which makes any significant change easier to manage.

   • Avoid drinks with caffeine to help you to sleep after you quit smoking (I show you how to curb your caffeine intake later in this chapter).

   • Satisfy your hunger with low-calorie beverages or snacks.

   • Relax yourself by exercising, taking a bath, or meditating.

   • Treat any cough with cough drops or hard candy.

2. **Benefit from the support of friends and loved ones.**

   Let everyone know you're quitting and ask for help, especially by not smoking in your presence. Even better, ask them to stop with you.

   Use individual or group counseling to support you. This may mean talking to someone several times a day when you're trying to quit. Check with your doctor or other healthcare provider for ideas that she may have to help you.

3. **Use new skills to handle problems that arise.**

Find enjoyable distractions (like exercise, reading a good book or watching a good movie) that substitute for the urge to smoke.

Stop activities that you combine with smoking (like an alcoholic drink or coffee, the morning break, or whatever you know to be a smoking trigger).

Change your routine to emphasize the lifestyle change. For example, go for a short walk first thing in the morning instead of lighting up.

Before you stop:

- Switch to a brand that you don't like that's low nicotine.
- Smoke only half the cigarette.
- Limit yourself to an increasingly smaller fixed number of cigarettes daily.
- After you get down to seven or less, set a quit date.
- Drink plenty of noncaloric fluids such as water.

4. **Make use of the medications that have proven to be effective in helping a person quit.**

Ask your doctor about nicotine replacement therapy and smoking cessation aids, which I discuss in more detail in the next section.

5. **Prepare for relapses.**

Everyone who has successfully quit smoking has probably done it on the second, third, or fourth try. Giving yourself another chance to succeed if your plan has a glitch is essential. A relapse usually occurs within the first three months. Meanwhile, you can avoid the situations where relapse is most likely:

- Try not to drink alcohol, which can lessen your control. (I discuss methods for avoiding alcohol later in this chapter.)
- Stay away from smokers. You don't even want a whiff of smoke.
- Don't return to smoking just because you gain weight. You can lose it sooner or later.
- Don't treat your nervousness, depression, or anxiety with a cigarette.

If you relapse, begin the process of quitting again as soon as possible. The less you smoke before beginning again, the easier it will be to quit again. Try to recognize the situations that blocked your previous attempts and avoid them the next time around.

Effective methods of quitting

Two effective methods for quitting smoking are nicotine replacement therapy and smoking cessation aids. You can buy some methods over-the-counter, but others require a prescription from your doctor. These are the details of each method:

✔ **Nicotine-replacement therapy:** The point of nicotine replacement therapy is to deliver small doses of nicotine to reduce the withdrawal symptoms. If you have high blood pressure associated with nicotine intake, plan to use this therapy as short a time as possible because nicotine in this form still raises your blood pressure. The therapy comes in five forms:

- **Nicotine gum,** available over-the-counter, comes in 2 mg and 4 mg strengths. As you chew, nicotine is released and absorbed by the membranes in the mouth. By reducing the number of pieces each day, you reach a day when you need none.

- **Nicotine lozenge,** a tablet that dissolves and delivers nicotine through the lining of your mouth, is also available in 2 and 4 mg doses.

- **Nicotine patches,** available both by prescription and over-the-counter, release nicotine gradually through the skin. They come in 15 mg strength or in varying doses that decline as withdrawal from tobacco continues.

  Note: People with allergies to adhesives have trouble with this method. Combining the gum or lozenges with the patches may work better than either alone, but be sure to get your doctor's approval before using both treatments together.

- **Nicotine nasal spray** is available by prescription only. You inhale it whenever you have an urge to smoke. People with a sinus condition find it difficult to use.

- **Nicotine inhalers,** available by prescription, deliver nicotine in a vapor into the mouth, where the membranes absorb it. The inhalant may irritate the mouth and throat.

✔ **Smoking-cessation aids:** These don't contain nicotine but do decrease withdrawal symptoms. New preparations seem to appear almost daily. Some examples include the following:

- *Bupropion SR,* trade name Zyban, is available by prescription and acts to disrupt the addictive power of nicotine. At a dose of 300 mg given as 150 mg twice daily, it effectiveness has been proven in large studies of smokers.

  A combination of bupropion and a nicotine-replacement aid (see the previous list) accomplished a much higher rate of quitting than either one did alone.

- *Varenicline,* trade name Chantix, available by prescription, acts within the brain to diminish the high from smoking and decrease withdrawal symptoms. The dose is 1 mg twice a day.

- Nicotine vaccine is a potential new treatment that prevents nicotine from getting to the brain. This will be available in the next year or two. A single vaccination is required.

Tapping into resources

With the availability of the World Wide Web, you have many resources to help you quit smoking at the peck of a key on your computer keyboard. If you're computer-challenged, you can access these resources by mail or telephone. Here are the best of the lot:

- **Agency for Healthcare Research and Quality** has smoking cessation guidelines and other materials for both physicians and the public available at 301-427-1364 or on the Web at www.ahrq.gov.

- **American Cancer Society** has many pamphlets and Web pages on quitting smoking as well as a bibliography of books and tapes on quitting available at 800-227-2345 or www.cancer.org.

- **American Lung Association** has both information and clinics to help you stop smoking available at 800-586-4872 or www.lungusa.org.

- **American Heart Association** provides information on smoking-cessation programs in schools, workplaces, and healthcare sites. To obtain, call 800-242-8721 or visit the Internet at www.americanheart.org.

- **National Cancer Institute** (NCI) is a division of the National Institutes of Health. The NCI researches quitting smoking, promotes programs to decrease the impact of smoking on health, and publishes materials on the Internet and in hard copy with tips on quitting and avoiding second-hand smoke. The NCI supports the Cancer Information Service from which these materials are available at 800-4-Cancer. The Web address is cis.nci.nih.gov.

- **National Institute on Drug Abuse** (NIDA) is another part of the National Institutes of Health. It supports research on cigarettes and other sources of nicotine as an addictive drug. Fact sheets are available concerning drug abuse and addiction at 301-443-1124. The Web address is www.nida.nih.gov/.

- **Centers for Disease Control Tobacco Information and Prevention Source** has a database of smoking and health-related materials available at 800-232-4636 or on the Web at www.cdc.gov/tobacco.

- **Nicotine Anonymous** is a 12-step program. To find out more, call 415-750-0328 or visit the Internet at www.nicotine-anonymous.org.

Relating Alcohol to High Blood Pressure

This section tackles the second-most lethal substance you can put into your body: alcohol. Or maybe it's the *most* lethal. I guess it depends on whether you're looking at your lungs or your liver! In this section, I address men who drink more than two glasses of wine a day and more than ten glasses a week and women who drink more than a glass of wine a day and five a week.

Simply put, alcohol raises blood pressure. A comparison of the blood pressure of heavy drinkers (see the previous paragraph) with moderate and nondrinkers shows that alcohol does indeed raise blood pressure. When nondrinkers do drink alcohol, their blood pressure rises, and when heavy drinkers stop drinking, their blood pressure falls.

Abruptly stopping alcohol may cause a rise in blood pressure, so a doctor must carefully monitor this change.

Drinking large quantities of alcohol in one sitting (or standing, depending on the location!) also raises blood pressure, but it returns to normal if the drinking doesn't continue. However, an individual who drinks excessively for extended periods of time has a persistent increase in blood pressure. The longer a person drinks, the higher the blood pressure; the more a person drinks, the higher the blood pressure. In this case, the double negative does not create a positive!

Eighty to ninety-five percent of alcoholics smoke cigarettes. I want to emphasize that eliminating the power of one habit goes a long way towards eliminating the power of the other. Cigarettes and alcohol may go together like Will and Grace, but smoking and drinking isn't graceful or charming.

Surveying the symptoms of alcoholism

Alcoholism, the habitual or compulsive consumption of alcoholic liquor to excess, is an inherited physical abnormality, an inborn condition related to a certain type of body chemistry. Alcoholism is *not* a moral weakness.

A major medical consequence of alcoholism is a person's much greater risk for brain attacks. A study in *Annals of Internal Medicine* (January 2006) showed that drinking more than two glasses of wine or the equivalent on a daily basis led to a considerable increase in brain attacks. (See Chapter 7 for more information about brain attacks.)

If you're taking medication for high blood pressure and drinking heavily, you need to determine whether you're an alcoholic in order to clarify the role of your drinking in your blood pressure. You may be an alcoholic if you answer "Yes" to two or more of the following questions: Have you . . .

- ✔ Tried to reduce your drinking?
- ✔ Felt angry when someone talked to you about your drinking?
- ✔ Felt guilty about drinking?
- ✔ Used alcohol in the morning to *start the day* and settle your nerves?

The dire effects of demon drink

Endorphins, chemicals in the brain, are internal pleasure givers. The brain increases its release of endorphins when you drink alcohol. Habit-forming drugs like heroin also stimulate increased production of endorphins, creating a feeling of euphoria. Although alcoholics require more alcohol than a heroin addict requires heroin to get the same high, most people feel high at a blood level of 0.05 percent alcohol. The intoxication is severe at 0.2 percent blood level, and at 0.3 percent, the drinker may be in a coma. Death may occur when the level is 0.35 percent or higher.

Another way to determine whether you're an alcoholic is to count the number of drinks that you consume in a week. (A drink is a 12-ounce bottle of beer, 5 ounces of wine, or 1½ ounces of hard liquor.) Alcoholic men usually consume 15 or more drinks per week, and alcoholic women consume 12 or more. Those who consume more than five drinks in one sitting at least once a week are also considered alcoholics. Usually, alcoholics also . . .

- ✔ **Crave alcohol.** They have a strong need to drink.
- ✔ **Lose control when they drink.** They can't stop after they start.
- ✔ **Have a physical dependence on alcohol.** They have withdrawal symptoms (such as nervousness, shakiness, headache, and sweating) when they don't drink.
- ✔ **Have a tolerance to alcohol.** They need more alcohol than a nonalcoholic individual to achieve the same level of inebriation.

Looking at who's drinking

According to the *Journal of Studies on Alcohol* (November 2001), alcohol use begins in high school even though it's illegal to drink alcohol before the age of 18 in some states and 21 in the rest. In any given month, probably 70 percent of high school seniors have had alcohol to drink.

In the United States, the prevalence of alcoholism is 10 to 15 people per 100, which translates to more than 25 million alcoholics. An additional 10 million are problem drinkers who may become alcoholics, and the number of male alcoholics is only slightly greater than the number of females.

Alcohol abuse costs the United States 175 billion dollars every year due to lost productivity, early death, medical treatment, and legal fees for all the problems alcoholics get themselves into (such as auto accidents, fights, unprotected sex, and so forth).

Understanding alcohol's medical consequences

Alcohol abuse can lead to two major, long-term medical problems:

- ✔ *Cirrhosis* (tissue scarring) of the liver with gastrointestinal bleeding, liver failure, and death
- ✔ Heart disease associated with high blood pressure

The following list of additional health consequences from excessive alcohol use is long. Unfortunately, you don't get just one or another of these complications, but all of them at the same time. The load is too heavy for anyone to bear, particularly for the elderly.

- ✔ Depression of the central nervous system with loss of ability to perform complex tasks like driving; decreased attention span and short-term memory; impaired motor coordination
- ✔ Degeneration of the brain with loss of coordination and emotional stability; nerve degeneration with severe pain
- ✔ Addiction to tranquilizers to treat the emotional instability
- ✔ Physical damage in motor-vehicle crashes
- ✔ Increased risk of suicide and homicide
- ✔ Increased risk of unplanned pregnancy and sexually transmitted diseases
- ✔ Giving birth to a baby with fetal-alcohol syndrome, stunted growth, mental retardation, and other abnormalities of the face and heart
- ✔ Poor nutrition from an irritated liver and intestinal tract, which produces heartburn, nausea, and gas
- ✔ Loss of sex drive
- ✔ Neglect of food intake and physical appearance
- ✔ Sleep loss
- ✔ Severe inflammation of the pancreas with severe abdominal pain and nausea
- ✔ Increased incidence of cancer

Cancers of the mouth, throat, and esophagus have a much greater occurrence rate among those who drink and smoke than among those who only drink or those who only smoke:

- ✔ A drinker is six times more likely to get mouth and throat cancer as compared to a nondrinker.

- ✔ A smoker is seven times more likely to get mouth and throat cancer as compared to a nonsmoker.

- ✔ The individual who drinks and smokes is 38 times more likely to have mouth and throat cancer than the individual who neither drinks nor smokes.

Undergoing treatment

All the medical consequences of alcoholism (except cirrhosis of the liver, which is irreversible) start to reverse after you give up alcohol, particularly (for the purposes of this book) the blood pressure. In addition, you may regain your job, your family, other loved ones, and your self-respect.

Through the years, the study of alcoholism and its treatment has proven useful in many ways. Most importantly, we now know that the more help the alcoholic gets and uses, the greater his chance for prolonged sobriety. Statistics that support this philosophy include the following:

- ✔ Only 4 percent of alcoholics who try quitting on their own are sober after a year.

- ✔ 50 percent of alcoholics who go through treatment are sober after a year.

- ✔ 70 percent of alcoholics who go through treatment and regularly attend *Alcoholics Anonymous* (AA; see the later section "Alcoholics Anonymous") are sober after a year.

- ✔ 90 percent of alcoholics who go through treatment, attend AA meetings, and go to aftercare (self-help groups and individual therapy sessions) once a week are sober after one year.

Treatment and aftercare are undoubtedly valid and important. Treatment consists of three steps: a brief intervention during which the alcoholic is convinced to undergo therapy to stop drinking; a period of total abstinence from alcohol *(detoxification);* and finally, sessions that help the alcoholic develop techniques to keep her sober for the rest of her life. These techniques include drugs and AA.

The intervention

An intervention is recognized as the best way to help everyone affected by the person's drinking. It has two goals: first, to help the person who drinks excessively to stop; second, to help his loved ones deal with the issues his drinking has created. Even if the drinker can't be helped, the other people benefit greatly. These steps precede an intervention:

1. **Take care of yourself.**

   If you're the partner, child, parent, or employer of an alcoholic, first help yourself by going to Al-Anon (a support program similar to AA for the loved ones of the alcoholic). Second, get the support of a counselor who will provide a clear vision of the challenge and help you understand what *you* have to do to help the alcoholic.

2. **Use outside help for the alcoholic.**

   Find an addictions counselor to help you with the complicated process of getting your loved one or yourself off of alcohol. (For direction on finding a counselor, see the later section "Locating useful resources.")

3. **Create an intervention team.**

   This team consists of people who care about the alcoholic but whose lives have also been made miserable at times by the alcoholic's actions. The addictions counselor is an important part of the team. Each person puts in writing how the alcoholic has made his or her life miserable. They also tell the alcoholic to go to a treatment center and clearly indicate that they will no longer protect the alcoholic from her bad behaviors. Finally, they clearly explain how they will separate themselves from the alcoholic if treatment is not sought. For example, the spouse will leave the marriage.

When the alcoholic is sober, the team carries out the intervention in a controlled environment where she has to listen. The intervention continues until the alcoholic agrees to treatment or until the professional feels that nothing further can be done.

Detoxification

Detoxification means complete abstinence from alcohol. During this stage, the alcoholic must stop all drinking. Alcohol withdrawal consists of sweating, a rapid heartbeat, agitation, confusion, nausea and vomiting, and sometimes tremors or seizures. The alcoholic often becomes depressed. The symptoms may last three to seven days, but the doctor can treat them with medications.

During detoxification, the alcoholic should be evaluated for his addiction's medical consequences like liver disease and abnormalities of blood clotting. Alcoholics often show evidence of nutritional deficiencies and should be treated with vitamins, minerals, and a healthy, balanced diet.

Drug treatment

Total abstinence from alcohol is the goal of treatment. Absolutely no amount of alcohol, no matter how small, is acceptable for a recovering alcoholic.

The alcoholic enters a rehabilitation program of counseling, education, medical care, and nursing. Many of the people who help the alcoholic are recovering alcoholics, so they've *been there*.

Can moderate drinking benefit your health?

For years, people thought that a drink a day would keep the doctor away. And a number of studies have shown that people who drink moderately (no more than two drinks daily for men and one for women) have healthy improvements in their hearts and tend to live longer than people who don't drink at all.

But a more recent study of 5,500 men in Scotland published in the *British Medical Journal* (June 1999) showed that drinking two drinks daily led to a higher risk of dying from all causes as compared with drinking less alcohol. In another study from Harvard Medical School, researchers discovered a fat increase in the livers of men who ate well but who also had a daily dose of alcohol not large enough to cause inebriation. So a word to the wise: Don't start drinking just to obtain the medical *benefits* of alcohol.

The medications help prevent the alcoholic from returning to drinking or they block the effects of alcohol. The principal medications in current use are

- *Disulfiram* (brand name Antabuse): When mixed with alcohol, Antabuse triggers a severe hangover — headache, nausea, vomiting, increased blood pressure, and a rapid heartbeat. Note these cautions about this medication:

  - The person must be vigilant because many prepared foods like sauces and vinegars contain alcohol, which can set off a reaction.

  - It may continue to work up to two weeks after the individual quits taking it, and it shouldn't be used during pregnancy.

  - It interacts with certain other medications, especially blood thinners and anticonvulsants, so the doctor must be aware of the patient's other meds.

  - It can negatively affect mental illness and cause a severe allergic skin reaction.

  - It may reduce a person's sex drive and cause drowsiness (people who experience this reaction shouldn't use dangerous machinery or drive a car while on the drug).

  The patient takes the medication until he is in control of his drinking. This period may last months or even years.

- *Naltrexone* (brand name Revia): Naltrexone affects the pleasure chemicals that alcohol releases. The individual can no longer get high from alcohol, so there is little point in drinking. People don't become dependent on naltrexone and don't become euphoric when it's taken. The following cautions apply:

  - Naltrexone has been known to cause dizziness, headache, and weight loss, and there are cases of naltrexone abuse.

- Individuals with severe liver or kidney damage shouldn't take naltrexone.

- It doesn't make a person sober nor does it prevent a person from enjoying other sources of pleasure.

- Naltrexone blocks the effects of opiods such as morphine, so if the patient needs pain medication, it must be a non-narcotic.

Patients usually continue on naltrexone for three months if they successfully stop drinking.

✔ *Isradipine* (brand name Dynacirc): Although this drug was originally used for the treatment of high blood pressure, it helped those people who were drinking heavily by taking away the pleasure associated with drinking. The craving for alcohol rapidly diminishes and continues to decline as treatment continues. Cautions include the following:

- It may make a person feel light-headed and dizzy, so driving should be avoided until the patient's reaction to it is determined.

- It causes headaches and shouldn't be taken during pregnancy.

Using two of the drugs together may be more effective than one alone. Your doctor will make this determination.

These drugs don't work on a long-term basis without a treatment program such as AA.

Alcoholics Anonymous

A major step that an alcoholic can take is to join AA. Letting AA explain itself is probably best. I can tell you that more than 1 million recovered alcoholics are in AA in the United States and another million are in other countries. AA members meet in groups, large and small, to support one another. About 51,000 AA groups meet in the United States, and one is near you. Check online at www.alcoholics-anonymous.org or write to the main office to find a support group near you: Alcoholics Anonymous, Grand Central Station, P.O. Box 459, New York, NY 10163. You can also call 212-870-3400.

The support of AA is tremendously helpful for the alcoholic who utilizes it. A typical meeting consists of the group leader's description of the AA program followed by the personal histories of several members. A collection for the cost of the facilities and snacks is taken up and then the members leave or meet informally. All opinions and interpretations are those of the speaker himself. No one speaks for the whole group.

Alcoholics Anonymous provides an abundance of helpful literature — some is free and some has a nominal fee. The success of AA is based on the power of one recovering alcoholic to help an uncontrolled drinker by passing along information about his experiences and sobriety. The process works through the famous *Twelve Steps of Alcoholics Anonymous,* which can be found in any of their publications.

Locating useful resources

Numerous resources are available to the alcoholic who wishes to recover. The following list contains some of those resources. If you have access to the Internet, you can find tons of information. I have also added the phone number of each resource.

- **Al-Anon/Alateen** provides help for the loved ones of the alcoholic. It uses the principles of AA to help these people regain control over their lives and see what action they can take to help the alcoholic. Information on meetings, resources, and plenty of other help is available at www.al-anon.alateen.org on the Web. You can also call 757-563-1600.

- **Alcoholics Anonymous** has numerous sites on the Internet because so many of these groups dot the planet, but www.alcoholics-anonymous.org is the central Web site. Most of its publications are online along with directions to its groups worldwide. This is a key resource for anyone who lives with an alcoholic or is trying to quit alcohol. You can also call 212-870-3400. (See the previous section for more information about this group.)

- **American Council on Alcoholism** is a national nonprofit organization dedicated to addressing alcoholism as a treatable disease through identification, education, intervention, and referral. It has useful links to sites concerning college drinking, drunk driving, general information on alcoholism, government resources, professional organizations that deal with alcoholism, treatment and recovery, and drugs that help. It also has a link to the Web sites of the alcohol industry. The council is on the Internet at www.aca-usa.org and answers any question about alcoholism. You can also call 800-527-5344.

- **Internet Alcohol Recovery Center** is a central source for information on every aspect of alcohol abuse and treatment. A service of the University of Pennsylvania Health System, it has links to numerous resources and is a great place to start your education (after you've read this book, of course). It has such useful features as a substance abuse library and a directory of treatment professionals and support groups. You can find them online at www.uphs.upenn.edu/recovery/index.html or call them at 215-248-6025.

- **Mothers Against Drunk Driving** is another nationwide organization that provides information. It has over 600 chapters in this country and is dedicated to finding effective solutions to drunk driving and underage driving. Find it at www.madd.org or by phone at 800-438-6233.

Getting High on Caffeine

Caffeine is a chemical compound in the leaves, seeds, and fruits of more than 63 plant species, but it most commonly comes from coffee and cocoa beans, cola nuts, and tea leaves. But coffee isn't the only source of caffeine — a can of cola contains 45 mg, green tea has 30 mg, an ounce of chocolate has 20 mg, and even Anacin comes in at 65 mg for two tablets.

Although the case against caffeine isn't nearly as tidy as the ones against tobacco and alcohol, caffeine in any form has been shown to temporarily raise blood pressure. A cup or two of coffee doesn't seem to be damaging over the long-term, but the tendency to drink multiple cups of *high-octane* (heavily caffeinated) coffee is a definite cause of persistently elevated blood pressure.

People who drink four to five cups of coffee daily have an increase in blood pressure of 5 mm Hg. (See Chapter 2 for more on blood pressure measurement.) If they continue to drink that same amount, the blood pressure may fall *if* they don't have high blood pressure already. However, if they do have high pressure, they may be more sensitive to the blood-pressure-raising effect of caffeine; this blood pressure rise is then sustained. The effect is particularly true of the elderly population.

A 5 mm Hg rise in blood pressure may sound trivial, but it results in a 21 percent rise in the incidence of heart disease (see Chapter 5) and a 34 percent increase in the incidence of brain attacks (see Chapter 7). In addition, when taken with alcohol or tobacco, which is so often the case, the combination greatly increases the blood-pressure-raising effect of those drugs.

Studies about the effect of caffeine on blood pressure continue to come in. In the November 2005 *Journal of the American Medical Association,* a study of more than 250,000 women found that those who drank the most caffeine-containing drinks (including coffee and sodas) tended to have the highest blood pressures.

Having a cup of coffee just before your blood pressure is measured is unwise. The acute elevation in blood pressure may convince your doctor that you have sustained high blood pressure.

Knowing how much is too much

The daily recommended maximum amount of caffeine is 300 mg, and an ordinary cup of coffee (5 ounces) has 100 mg of caffeine. However:

✔ A short (8-ounce) cup of coffee at a nice café or fancy coffee shop contains 250 mg, more than double the amount of that ordinary cup.

✔ A tall (12-ounce) cup of coffee from the same shop is 375 mg, nearly four times that ordinary cup.

✔ A coffee grande (16 ounces) packs 550 mg, more than five times the punch.

You can see where a few cups of coffee can quickly add up to much more than each day's recommended maximum.

Considering caffeine's health consequences

Caffeine is a mildly addictive drug. When a person stops drinking it, she has withdrawal symptoms such as:

✔ Feelings of sleepiness

✔ Feelings of being overtired

✔ A severe headache

But caffeine also has a number of potential medical consequences when a person consumes it in large doses (over 300 mg daily) over a period of years:

✔ *Osteoporosis* (thinning of the bone)

As a result of the urine-promoting effect of caffeine, the calcium that a body needs to build strong bones passes quickly into the urine. Women (and men) are encouraged to manage this problem by taking milk with the caffeine and getting extra calcium from other sources like dairy products or calcium pills.

✔ Infertility, birth defects, and miscarriages

✔ Heartburn and even ulcers due to increased stomach acid production

Who doesn't drink coffee with caffeine? Me. Several years ago, I stopped drinking caffeinated beverages and immediately stopped having abdominal pain; I've had none of those symptoms since then.

✔ Increased risk of heart disease when coffee is unfiltered (more frequent before 1975)

✔ Increased premenstrual pain and formation of breast lumps, but these are controversial findings

✔ Poor sleep quality and difficulty falling asleep

Caffeine can keep you awake, but it does *not* improve your performance of complex tasks.

Recognizing the gains in giving up caffeine

When you give up caffeine, you eliminate the chance of developing any of the conditions in the preceding section, you eliminate an unnecessary drug from your body, *and* you help keep your blood pressure under control. As a woman, you may greatly enhance your chance of becoming pregnant and having a healthy pregnancy and delivery.

Note: The coffee bean isn't a vegetable — no fair trying to get credit in the vegetable category of your DASH diet for consuming it.

Warning: You may become a coffee addict if you name your child *Mocha* and your dog *Java!*

Avoiding the beans, chocolate, and soda

If you consume no more than two cups of coffee daily, you should have no symptoms if you switch to decaffeinated drinks and avoid other sources of caffeine like chocolate. I was in that category when I gave up caffeine, yet I did go through a period of mild withdrawal symptoms (see the earlier section about these consequences).

For the person who consumes much more caffeine daily, the process of quitting may be more difficult. Here are some practical suggestions:

- ✔ Try to determine how much caffeine you're taking in each day. Check all foods and medications to make sure you're not missing an unexpected source.

- ✔ Reduce your intake and see how you feel as you withdraw.

- ✔ Gradually reduce your daily caffeine by 50 mg or so until you're free of it.

- ✔ Use exercise to give you the energy that you believe was coming from caffeine. (I discuss exercise in detail in Chapter 12.)

- ✔ Avoid the other habits such as smoking that go with drinking coffee.

- ✔ Ask the people you live and eat with to help you by reducing their caffeine intake. The improvement they feel will make them grateful.

Some pros and cons of caffeine

The final determination on all the effects of coffee, negative and positive, isn't in. Some studies indicate that coffee may protect against cancer of the large intestine and rectum. Others suggest that it may have a protective effect against the damage that alcohol does to the liver. Very careful future studies can show whether these theories are valid. Most recently, in the February 2006 *Diabetes Care,* a study of more than 88,000 women reported that the occurrence of diabetes was reduced among those who drank caffeinated or decaffeinated coffee.

But one proven, damaging consequence of caffeine is that it affects the woman who wants to become pregnant. Consuming more than three cups of caffeinated coffee each day reduces fertility. And the woman who is pregnant may deliver an underweight baby if she consumes more than three cups daily during her pregnancy. A few women who consumed enormous amounts of caffeine — 8 to 25 cups of coffee every day — delivered babies with birth defects.

Using resources

You can check a few Internet sites for the latest information on this controversial drug. These two are among the best:

- **Center for Science in the Public Interest** is a large Web source on a wide variety of topics, just as its title suggests. It also publishes the *Nutrition Action Healthletter.* Find any new information on the health effects of caffeine at www.cspinet.org or by phone at 202-332-9110.

- **Columbia University's Health Question & Answer Internet Service called "Go Ask Alice"** is one of the best university hospital sites on the Web for information on caffeine. The address is www.goaskalice.columbia.edu; no phone number is available.

Chapter 12

Lowering Blood Pressure with Exercise

*W*hen I see new patients with high blood pressure, I give them a bottle of pills right away. But the pills aren't for oral consumption. Instead, they're for dropping on the floor and picking up one at a time several times a day — a good start to an exercise program!

Of course, you need to make up your mind to exercise, but the benefits of a regular program can't be denied. Two significant effects are the following:

✔ Exercise can lower blood pressure — especially for people who have high blood pressure.

✔ Exercise causes weight reduction and weight loss maintenance, which also help to lower blood pressure.

In addition, an exercise test can help determine which people are likely to develop high blood pressure. People with an exaggerated rise in blood pressure during exercise are much more likely to develop sustained high blood pressure later in life. They need to be watched more carefully.

I asked a patient who refused to exercise whether it was because of ignorance or apathy. The patient replied, "I don't know, and I don't care." Read this chapter. Then if you don't exercise, at least it won't be because of ignorance.

Understanding the Benefits of Physical Activity

Exercise strengthens all the muscles involved in your body's movement. If you walk or jog, you strengthen your leg muscles. If you lift packages, you strengthen your arm muscles. Whatever the exercise, your heart muscles become stronger. At the same time, your body opens up your arteries to allow for more flow of nutrients into the tissues. The combination of a stronger, more efficient heart and more open blood vessels leads to lower blood pressure.

Lowering your blood pressure is a good enough reason to make exercise an important part of your lifestyle, but if you need more, check out this list for additional benefits from exercise:

- ✔ Improves your memory
- ✔ Reduces the risk of breast cancer and large intestinal cancer
- ✔ Lowers blood sugar, thus protecting you against diabetes
- ✔ Increases energy level
- ✔ Improves mood
- ✔ Makes you sexier
- ✔ Helps you sleep better
- ✔ Strengthens your bones
- ✔ Lowers bad cholesterol and raises good cholesterol

Need even more reasons? Pick up a copy of *Fitness For Dummies,* 3rd Edition, by Suzanne Schlosberg and Liz Neporent (Wiley), where you find 100 reasons to become fit.

Preparing for Exercise

Take these three important steps before you begin an exercise program:

1. **Determine your current physical condition to decide what type of exercise program is right for your fitness level.**

2. **Choose the exercises that you plan to make part of your program.**

3. **Get the right equipment.**

Checking your physical condition

When you know your beginning fitness level, you can chart your progress. One simple way to test your fitness level is to:

1. **Take your pulse.**

2. **Walk a mile.**

3. **Note how long it took you to walk and your pulse rate at the end of the mile.**

The time and your pulse give you a baseline for comparison as you improve.

To take your pulse: With your palm upward, place your index and middle finger over the wrist artery that's about ½ inch in from the outside of the wrist. (Don't use your thumb to feel because it has its own pulse and can confuse your count.) Count the number of beats for 15 seconds and multiply by four to get your one-minute pulse rate. (If you can't feel your pulse in the wrist, try feeling the pulse in your neck, where it's much stronger.)

Write down the number before you forget it! You can do this simple test about once a month and you'll be astounded at your progress as your pulse gets slower and slower — indicating a much more efficient heart.

If you haven't exercised for many years, don't start a program without some preparation. People over the age of 40 should talk to their doctor and have a physical examination. Your doctor may recommend an *exercise electrocardiogram,* better known as an *exercise test* or *stress test.* This test looks at the response of your heart to fairly vigorous exercise. If you get through an exercise electrocardiogram without problems such as chest pain, severe shortness of breath, or changes in your electrocardiogram, you're probably in good enough shape to begin an exercise program.

Ask your doctor to help you map out an exercise plan that can strengthen your heart and prevent high blood pressure. If you already have high blood pressure, discuss a plan that can help lower your blood pressure to an agreeable level.

When you begin your exercise program, keep these facts in mind:

✔ **Start slowly and build up over time.** You don't need to rush to get to a certain level of exercise by a certain date. Gradually work your way along until you achieve your goal.

✔ **You don't need to go farther and faster after you reach a level of fitness that affects your blood pressure.** That desired fitness level may lower your blood pressure by as much as 10 millimeters of mercury systolic (see Chapter 2 for more about blood pressure measurement), which is just as good as most pills can accomplish.

If you're really enjoying the exercise and want to rev it up, that's up to you — but going farther and faster won't lower your blood pressure any more.

✔ **People with high blood pressure have a post-exercise fall in blood pressure that may last seven or eight hours.** Therefore, *daily* exercise can have a much more profound effect on your blood pressure than exercising only three or four times a week.

Choosing exercises

For maximum fitness, most exercise programs combine two types of exercises: aerobic and anaerobic.

✔ **Aerobic** means *with oxygen*. During aerobic exercise, the body uses oxygen to help provide energy. Aerobic activity can be sustained for more than a few minutes, and it involves major groups of muscles (particularly the legs but also the arms if you can't use your legs). Activities such as walking, running, cycling, tennis, basketball, and so forth make your heart pump faster during the exercise.

✔ **Anaerobic** means *without oxygen*. Anaerobic exercises are very intense, so they can't be sustained for very long. Examples are lifting heavy weights and doing the 100-yard dash. They depend on sources of energy that are already available (like glucose in your muscle).

Engaging in a regular aerobic exercise program can, over time, lower your blood pressure up to 10 millimeters of mercury systolic and enable you to get off a blood pressure medication. In contrast, anaerobic exercises, although great for increasing the strength of individual muscles, don't go on long enough to improve heart function or lower your blood pressure. But a program of both aerobic and anaerobic exercises gives you the best of both worlds — lower blood pressure and stronger muscles. (See the "Exercising for Strength" section later in this chapter for practical anaerobic exercise ideas.)

Stepping up to a multilevel walking program

The range of aerobic exercise choices is limitless. Mix it up a bit. Play tennis several days a week and do something else, perhaps walking, the other days. Walking is the exercise that almost everybody can do; you don't have to belong to a special club, and, unless you live in an area that has snow a good portion of the year, you can walk outside most any day — even in the rain. (Use an umbrella; you can't melt.) You can easily walk alone, but walking with a friend makes the activity more pleasant and also allows you to encourage each other to stay committed.

Table 12-1 outlines a walking program that starts slowly; most people can complete Level 1 without a great deal of difficulty. (If the distance is too great for you, begin with half the distance.) When you can accomplish the goals of one level once a day for seven days, you're ready to move to the next level.

If you did the test that I describe earlier in "Checking your physical condition," you already know how fast you can walk a mile. Start at that level, not a slower one, and build from there. If you didn't do a fitness test, walk a mile and check your time. Begin the seven days at that level.

Table 12-1 breaks the walking program into 15 levels so you can work your way up to a desired level of fitness to lower your blood pressure.

Table 12-1	Walking Program to Achieve Lower Blood Pressure	
Level	*Distance (in Miles)*	*Time (in Minutes)*
1	1	30
2	1	28
3	1	26
4	1	24
5	1	22
6	1	20
7	1½	32
8	1½	31
9	1½	30
10	1½	29
11	1½	28
12	1½	27
13	1½	26
14	1½	25
15	1½	24

Thirty minutes a day is the minimum recommended length of exercise. When you reach Level 15 (or 1⅝ miles in 30 minutes), you can stay there permanently. It will make a significant difference in your blood pressure as well as other aspects of your health. Surely you can spare half an hour daily to make a huge impact on your health.

Walking 10,000 steps every day

An alternative to the 15-level program is to walk 10,000 steps a day, which may be easier because you get constant feedback. Use a *pedometer,* a device you wear on your waist, to count your steps. Keep track of your daily steps for a week to get your average daily steps. Then try to increase your steps by 500 daily. When you've gone seven days at this new level, go for another 500. Keep increasing until you've reached 10,000 steps a day.

At 10,000, you're walking about five miles. "Impossible!" you say. Isn't it amazing what you can do when you make up your mind?

Pedometers are available at sports stores, but you can find some of the best and most reliable at www.accusplit.com. For more help with this program, go to www.thewalkingsite.com/10000steps.html.

If you really want to turn your walking into fun and education, go to http://walking.about.com/cs/beginners/1/blwebwalkingadt.htm for the American Discovery Trail, a virtual tour across the country with links to all the interesting sights along the way. You can *walk* from Cape Henlopen State Park in Delaware to Point Reyes National Seashore in California by converting your daily steps to miles (simply eliminate the last two digits; for example, 10,000 steps becomes 100 miles). The Web site tells you what you *see* as you add miles each day. Who knows — you may decide to do it for real.

Choosing other aerobic activities

Walking is great exercise and certainly one of the simplest, but don't feel like you *have to* walk to enjoy the pressure-lowering effects of exercise. If you prefer other types of aerobically effective activities, feel free! Just make sure you can do them *and* stick with them. Table 12-2 lists some of those activities. In addition, consider racquetball, squash, handball, rowing, judo, karate, social dancing, and singles tennis. People from different cultures may also have different exercises that they particularly like such as soccer, rugby, and cricket. *What* you do doesn't really matter; but you have to do *something*.

Getting the right equipment

If you plan to engage in an exercise that may cause friction in your joints like walking and jogging, get the best footwear you can afford. Some of the sneakers available today seem awfully pricey, but when you consider what you save in the *long run* (pun intended) in health costs, then they're well worth the price.

Try to find a store where the staff is knowledgeable about shoe needs, perhaps one that caters to runners and walkers.

Make sure you have the right clothes for your exercise. Dressing in layers is a good idea because you can remove clothing as you heat up. Some sports clothes are better than others because they *sweat,* allowing your perspiration to pass through and evaporate rather than sticking to your body. This process cools you off and helps you to feel less wet as you exercise. Polyesters work well, but cotton absorbs the moisture and holds it against your skin. For cooler weather, choose an outer layer that repels wind and rain but allows sweat to pass through.

If you choose to do plenty of biking, make sure you have a bike suitable for the terrain. Bikes that are good for flat streets are very different from mountain bikes. Even the tires are different. If you want to limit yourself to an indoor stationary cycle, make sure the quality is good. Plenty of resources such as *Consumer Reports* magazine are available to guide your decision. You can also find help on the Internet. Two excellent resources are Road Bike Review at www.roadbikereview.com and Mountain Bike Review at www.mtbr.com.

Knowing the Right Levels of Exercise

Want to know whether your exercise is making a difference in your fitness? You could do a fitness test each time you exercise. But because you don't make huge strides each time, you'd definitely be disappointed. In the past, fitness advisors suggested measuring your heart rate during exercise. If your pulse was in the *training* range, it was fast enough to improve your fitness but not too fast to overexert your heart. But today's research shows that the concept of the training range is probably not useful.

Today's research shows that people can exercise with a faster pulse than their training range and benefit from it by rating their physical activity of choice according to the *Perceived Exertion Scale* (which compares favorably with the pulse and consumption of oxygen, two measures known to correlate with fitness). The scale helps people determine whether an activity is making a difference in their fitness, and these are the basics:

- ✔ You rate the degree of your exertion while performing a certain activity from *very, very light* to *very, very hard* — according to your personal physical ability level.

- ✔ In-between levels are *very light, fairly light, somewhat hard, hard, very hard,* and *extremely hard.*

  - *Very light* is like walking slowly for several minutes.

  - *Fairly light* means you're breathing harder but can continue.

- *Somewhat hard* exercise is getting a little difficult but still feels okay to continue.

- *Hard* means you're starting to have trouble breathing; speaking is difficult.

- *Very hard* exercise is difficult to continue, so you have to push yourself; you're very tired and have trouble talking comfortably.

- *Extremely hard* exercise is the most difficult you have ever tried.

✔ The *very hard* level of exercise is most beneficial.

✔ As your fitness level increases, your definition of *very hard* changes. What was once *very hard* may become *fairly light*.

Exercise is beneficial for every stage of high blood pressure (see Chapter 2 for details about these stages). However, doctors generally recommend that people with blood pressure in the higher stage 2 (greater than 160 systolic and 100 diastolic) exercise at a slightly lower level than stage 1 patients. Referring to the Perceived Exertion Scale, stage 2 patients should work at the *somewhat hard* instead of the *very hard* level.

To learn more about the Perceived Exertion Scale, check out `www.cdc.gov/ nccdphp/dnpa/physical/measuring/perceived_exertion.htm` and `www.pponline.co.uk/encyc/1020.htm` on the Web.

Exercising to Lose Weight

Exercise can help you lose weight, but you need to exercise at least 90 minutes six days a week. (To maintain a weight loss, you need to do 60 minutes daily; to get into good physical shape and have an effect on your blood pressure, you need at least 30 minutes a day.)

The exercise doesn't have to be continuous. Three ten-minute sessions are as good as 30 uninterrupted minutes.

A kilocalorie is the amount of energy needed to raise the temperature of a kilogram of water 1 degree centigrade, and a pound of fat contains 3,500 *kilocalories* (kcals). So, to lose a pound of fat, you must use (burn, exercise, whatever) at least 3,500 kilocalories more than you eat. For example, if you eat 2,000 kilocalories each day to maintain your weight, you can lose 1 pound in seven days by using 500 kilocalories more each day than usual ($500 \times 7 = 3,500$). Doing only 250 kilocalories of extra exercise takes 14 days to lose the same pound. Walking an hour each day burns 4 kilocalories per minute, 240 kilocalories in all.

Table 12-2 shows the number of kilocalories that you burn doing several different kinds of exercise for 30, 45, or 60 minutes.

Table 12-2	Kilocalories Burned Doing Various Exercises		
Activity	*30 Minutes*	*45 Minutes*	*60 Minutes*
Doubles tennis	85	128	170
Walking a 20-min mile on flat surface	120	180	240
Water aerobics	140	210	280
Walking a 15-min mile on flat surface	146	219	292
Walking a 20-min mile uphill	162	243	324
Golf (carrying your bag)	174	261	348
Walking a 15-min mile uphill	206	309	412
Swimming	250	375	500
Basketball	282	423	564
Bicycling (12 mph)	283	425	566
Cross-country skiing	291	438	583
Aerobic dance	342	513	684
Running 10-min miles	365	549	732

Exercising for Strength

A complete exercise program includes aerobic exercises to lower your blood pressure and anaerobic exercises to strengthen your muscles. (See the earlier section "Choosing exercises" for more about aerobic activities.) Strengthening your muscles allows you to do more aerobic exercise as well as improve your balance. To add an anaerobic element to your workout, get yourself some *dumbbells* of various weights and some *barbells,* to which you can add more weight as you get stronger. Use dumbbells of no more than 5 to 10 pounds when you start. In just a few days, those weights will feel light.

If you have high blood pressure, use weights that allow you to do many repetitions of an exercise instead of a few extreme lifts with very large weights. Extreme lifting may suddenly raise your blood pressure to unacceptable levels.

A weight-lifting program requires no more than 15 minutes of your time about five days a week. Do it for two days, skip a day, do it for another three days, skip a day, then back to two days, and so on. These breaks allow your muscles to recover between exercise workouts.

If you stick to the simple program in the following sections, you'll be amazed and delighted at the rapid progress you make in body strength, increased fitness, and increased self-assurance. Just be sure to increase the weights as they become easier to lift so you continue reaping the rewards. Among other benefits, weight lifting helps you

- Keep your bones stronger
- Prevent injuries by improving balance
- Look better
- Speed up your metabolism

You can expect to increase your muscle strength 7 to 40 percent with ten weeks of training.

Upper-body exercises

The following list describes seven exercises that you can do in 15 minutes to improve your upper-body strength. Simply do 15 repetitions of each exercise and move on to the next. Each series of 15 repetitions of seven exercises is called a *circuit*. Do two circuits without stopping each time that you exercise. Start with an amount of weight that allows you to complete the 15 repetitions. If you can't do 15, you're using too much weight and overexerting yourself.

- **Shoulder press:** Stand with your feet shoulder-width apart and knees slightly bent. With dumbbells in each hand, start with your hands next to your shoulders facing inward. Raise the dumbbells over your head until your arms are straight. Bring the weights back down to the starting position, palms facing each other.
- **Lateral raise:** Hold a dumbbell in each hand by your sides, palms facing each other. Raise the dumbbells out to the sides, keeping your arms straight (but don't lock your elbows) and your palms facing the floor, until they're above your head. Return them to the starting position.

✔ **Bent-over rowing:** Bend from the waist, keeping your knees slightly bent, until your upper body is parallel with the floor. With a dumbbell in each hand and your arms hanging straight down, slowly raise the dumbbells out to the side until they're in line with your shoulders. Lower them again.

✔ **Good mornings:** Stand straight, holding a single dumbbell with both hands over your head. Keeping your arms straight over your head, bend from the waist until your torso and arms are parallel with the floor. Then raise yourself to the starting point.

✔ **Flys:** Lie on your back with one dumbbell in each hand and your arms opened out to each side at shoulder height. Slowly raise the dumbbells in over your body until they touch above your chest. Slowly lower them back to the starting position.

✔ **Pullovers:** Lie on your back with your knees bent, holding one dumbbell with both hands above your chest. Lower the dumbbell back over your head until it touches the floor. Then raise it back over your chest.

✔ **Curls:** Stand straight, holding a barbell in each hand in front of you. With your palms facing up, slowly bend your elbows until your hands are shoulder height. Lower them back slowly to the starting position.

Evaluating the strength of your upper and lower body

Push-ups are a good way to evaluate your upper-body strength. To do a push-up:

1. Lie face down on the floor with your palms about shoulder-width apart.

2. Push yourself up off the floor, straightening your arms and keeping your back and legs straight.

3. Lower yourself until your chest just touches the floor, but don't let your weight rest on the floor.

4. Continue Steps 2 and 3 until you grow too tired to do any more, keeping track of how many you can do.

Squats are good evaluators of your lower-body strength. To do a squat:

1. Stand up straight with your arms by your sides and legs about shoulder-width apart.

2. Begin to bend your knees as you raise your arms to a horizontal position at your sides.

3. When your thighs are parallel with the ground, go back up again.

4. Continue Steps 2 and 3 until you grow too tired to do any more, keeping track of how many you can do.

Save these numbers for future comparison. Test yourself at intervals of four to six weeks to keep track of your progress and to keep yourself motivated in your exercise program.

Leg-strengthening exercises

A couple of standard exercises for strengthening leg muscles, repeated 15 times each for two sets, include the following:

- ✔ **Lunge:** Stand straight with your feet about shoulder-width apart. Hold a light dumbbell in each hand, palms facing your body. Take a long step forward with the right foot and bend the right leg until your thigh is parallel with the ground. Hold the position a second, and then step back and straighten your leg. Lunge forward with the other leg.

- ✔ **Squat:** Stand straight with your feet hip-width apart. Place a barbell containing light weights behind your neck and hold it with your hands. Bend your knees slowly and squat until your thighs are parallel with the ground. Pause, and then rise to the standing position.

Lowering Your Blood Pressure with Alternative Therapies

Although aerobic exercise is extremely helpful for lowering blood pressure, other disciplines *(alternative therapies)* can help accomplish this goal as well. When combined with exercise, the result can be significant. I can't vouch for the value of each form for treating high blood pressure, but people can follow many different paths toward controlling their blood pressure. Perhaps one of these methods will appeal to you, and you can utilize it to save yourself from years of medical problems and expenses related to high blood pressure (not to mention all the other diseases waiting out there for patients with high blood pressure).

Yoga, meditation, hypnosis, and biofeedback are the most useful forms of alternative therapy for high blood pressure, but by no means are they the only forms. Holistic Online (www.holisticonline.com) lists no fewer than 20 different forms of alternative medicine. You may want to consider trying one or several of these practices. (They have some overlap in their effects, but each one is distinctive enough to have a following of devotees.)

Yoga

Yoga is a series of postures and breathing exercises developed in India over 5,000 years ago as a way to achieve *union (yoga)* with the *divine consciousness*. Today, people often practice yoga as a way of improving their health and well-being without putting an emphasis on yoga's religious side. Yoga attempts to unite your body and your mind so your mind can function better in a more healthy body. Numerous studies have shown that yoga can lower blood pressure. A July 2006 article in the *Clinical Journal of Sports Medicine* points out the positive effect of yoga on blood pressure. This effect persists as long as the practice continues, and it often disappears if the individual stops practicing yoga.

Over its 5,000-years existence, yoga has evolved in many directions as teachers developed their different philosophies. As a result, yoga has eight main branches. *Hatha yoga,* the most popular branch, emphasizes physical fitness more than the others do. But this branch subscribes to plenty of meditation and spiritualism as well.

 An excellent source of information about all aspects of yoga is *Yoga For Dummies* by Georg Feuerstein and Larry Payne (Wiley). I highly recommend it. The Internet also offers many excellent yoga sites. The following are two of the best:

- ✔ **The Yoga Site** (www.yogasite.com) can answer all your questions and direct you to many other useful sites.

- ✔ **The Yoga Journal** (www.yogajournal.com) provides numerous articles concerning the world of yoga.

Meditation

Meditation involves concentrating on an object, a sound, a word, or the breath in order to diminish random thoughts. The result is a calmer, more peaceful mind. Meditation doesn't involve specific body postures like yoga does, but some aspects of yoga involve meditation, particularly the awareness of the breathing.

Meditation may be the best studied of the various forms of relaxation. Articles in the May 2005 *American Journal of Hypertension* and the January 2005 *American Journal of Cardiology* compare meditation with other forms of relaxation and find that the effect of meditation is significant in lowering blood pressure, much better than muscle relaxation and mental relaxation. Many clinical studies have shown that meditation can lower blood pressure and keep it down as long as the practice is continued.

 Just like yoga, meditation has gone in different directions over the years. The most popular form is *Transcendental Meditation.* You can find out much more about this technique by obtaining (you guessed it) *Meditation For Dummies* by Stephan Bodian (Wiley). Some of the best Internet resources on meditation are the following:

- ✔ **Learning Meditation** (www.learningmeditation.com) is an award-winning site that explains meditation and how to use it in your daily life to find more calm and serenity. The author of this site actually prefers the term *conscious relaxation* or *chosen relaxation* to *meditation*. The site is well done, and I highly recommend it.

- ✔ **Holistic Online** (www.holisticonline.com) describes just about every kind of alternative therapy that exists, including meditation and even humor therapy. If meditation isn't what you're looking for, the site probably has something else that you can get into.

Hypnosis

Hypnosis is a form of *guided meditation* (guided by another person or one-self) that slows down the brain and allows the hypnotized person to respond, within limitations, to the suggestions of the hypnotist. The definition often describes a sleeplike state, but practitioners insist that the hypnotized person isn't asleep because she can hear and respond. *Note:* A hypnotized person won't do anything she doesn't want to do.

Studies show that hypnosis can lower mildly elevated blood pressure when appropriate relaxation instructions are given. People can hypnotize them-selves and control blood pressure effectively.

You can find some excellent information on hypnosis on the Internet (what a surprise!). The following Web sites appear to have some very useful and valid information:

- ✔ **Hypnosis.com** (www.hypnosis.com) has frequently asked questions that provide a clear explanation of hypnosis and what it can do for you. It clears up many myths about this useful therapy, particularly the myth that, under its influence, you can be induced to do something you would never do ordinarily.

- ✔ **The American Society of Clinical Hypnosis** (www.asch.net) can help you find a therapist, and it explains a hypnotist's certification. The site directs you to videos and books that help you get a clearer picture of hypnosis.

Biofeedback

Biofeedback is a technique developed in the late 1960s in which you train your-self to alter an *involuntary function* (like heart rate, body temperature, or in your case, blood pressure) with the aid of a *biofeedback machine*. (Biofeedback machines detect a person's internal bodily functions so the functions can be altered.)

For example, one biofeedback machine picks up electrical signals from muscles and translates them into a flashing light. In order to reduce the tension in her muscles, the person using the machine first figures out how to slow down the flashes of light. After awhile, she no longer needs the machine to relax; she simply uses the methods she discovered with the machine.

Various kinds of equipment are available for biofeedback, and numerous Internet sites can help you find them. One of these sites is the Holistic Online site (www.holisticonline.com), which I list earlier in the "Meditation" section. A couple of other valuable sites are as follows:

- ✔ **The Association for Applied Psychophysiology and Biofeedback** (www.aapb.org) contains answers to your questions as well as a list of practitioners, a bookstore for relevant books, and links to more information.

- ✔ **The Biofeedback Network** (www.biofeedback.net) is an online source for equipment, information, links, practitioners, and biofeedback centers. Its mission is to provide "Quality On-line Biofeedback Resources to the world biofeedback community." That community may include you.

Chapter 13

Adding Drug Therapy

When I reviewed a recent publication on drug treatments for high blood pressure, I came to a list of current drugs — no fewer than 72 in six different classes. Surely, a doctor can find one or more that are perfect for you.

Not so fast! First, have you maximized the lifestyle changes that lower blood pressure without drugs, as I discuss in Chapters 8 through 12? If you can say, "Yes!" to this question but your blood pressure is still elevated, ask your doctor about prescribing one of the drugs in this chapter. However, if you answered "No" to my question about lifestyle changes, I strongly suggest you go back and do what you can to reduce your blood pressure without drugs.

The drug choices are almost limitless, but don't let every new drug that comes along fool you. Glitzy TV and radio commercials and magazine ads are designed to manipulate your imagination, suggesting that your life can be a bowl of cherries if you pop a new drug. Keep in mind:

✔ Some drugs are inappropriate for some people with high blood pressure.

✔ Some drugs may have miserable side effects that affect you and just a few other people.

✔ If you already take a prescription medicine, adding another drug can create a problem because of the drug interactions that change the effect of each one.

In this chapter, I first answer general questions about drugs and then take up the individual drug classes and the drugs within them. You need to know how these drugs act, how long they act, what the side effects are, what dosages to take, how they interact with other medications, and what physical limits preclude their use.

As I point out elsewhere in this book, despite the availability of excellent drugs, only about 25 percent of all people with high blood pressure control it. This brings up the problem of compliance. Taking your drug the first weeks or months after your doctor has made a diagnosis of high blood pressure is easy, but what about the years after that? As you continue to suffer from high blood pressure — the silent killer — will you lose your resolve to control it? After all, you may feel fine, and you may not see your doctor for six months or a year.

Of course, losing your resolve to control your blood pressure would be a serious mistake. One way to stay motivated is to understand your medication completely and the reasons you're taking it — that's my goal with the high level of detail in this chapter.

Because you may be taking only one or two of the many drugs in this chapter, you may want to confine your review to those drugs. But at least check out the introductory remarks for each of the drug classes and take a look at the section "Choosing a Drug" to make sure you're on the right track. Your doctor may find that you'd do much better with a prescription from another class. In that case, being an informed consumer can put you in a position to ask your doctor intelligent questions.

Your pharmacist can be a great resource for drug information. Also, a publication called the *Physicians' Desk Reference* (PDR) is available in most doctors' offices and hospital libraries and has the latest information about all drugs. ***Note:*** All the information in it comes from the drug companies.

Want another resource? A site called *Epocrates* at www.epocrates.com has a more balanced database of all prescription drugs that you can download to your computer or personal digital assistant (PDA). It's constantly updated so you stay in touch with the latest drug treatments.

Establishing Drug Characteristics

High blood pressure medications have different characteristics and features — some may be beneficial, but others may be detrimental to you. Be sure you find out about a medication's main features before you chase a new pill down with a glass of water.

How effective is it?

Doctors like to have proof in the form of medical studies that the drugs are effective and work as advertised. But this process takes ten years or more after a drug has been approved by the Food and Drug Administration (FDA) and comes onto the market, and many of the drugs in this chapter have been around for only a few years. Drug manufacturers often claim that a new drug in the same class as a proven old drug should work the same. However, the new drug may produce side effects that only become apparent after years of use on thousands of people. So you always have to be wary.

How much can it lower blood pressure as compared to another drug?

Up to a certain point, the lower the blood pressure, the better off the patient. However, several studies have shown that when the blood pressure goes below a certain level (which is not the same for each person), the risk of a heart attack increases (possibly because the pressure is so low that not enough blood is reaching the heart muscle). None of the commonly used drugs, when used alone, lower the blood pressure past that point. But of the various classes, *thiazide diuretics* lower the systolic blood pressure more than the others. (It lowers the diastolic blood pressure about the same as other drugs.) See Chapter 2 for details on diastolic and systolic blood pressure.

Do drugs that lower blood pressure to the same extent have the same effect on disease and death?

Thiazide diuretics lower blood pressure more than the other classes of commonly used drugs.

It's natural to assume that a blood-pressure-lowering drug prevents the long-term consequences of high blood pressure, but this isn't necessarily the case. Nevertheless, the old standards, especially the thiazide diuretics, have proven effective (though not in all circumstances) against long-term consequences.

In fact, the evidence shows that even when a drug other than a thiazide diuretic lowers the blood pressure to the same extent, thiazides prevent disease and death more than other blood-pressure-lowering drugs. If you've concluded that I have a definite preference for thiazide diuretics as initial drug treatment for high blood pressure, you're right.

Presenting the Classes of Drugs

Drugs that lower blood pressure are divided into several classes: diuretics, drugs that act on the nervous system, vasodilators, calcium channel blocking agents, angiotensin-converting enzyme inhibitors, and angiotensin II receptor blockers. Each class works by a different mechanism, and I discuss those later in this chapter.

I categorize the drugs in this chapter by the *way* they lower blood pressure, and I mention all the drugs currently available in each class because your doctor may have a preference for one or another. The drugs are referred to by their generic names, that is, their official chemical designations.

Many manufacturers make the same drug and then give it their own brand name. I list those brand names in parentheses after the generic names throughout the chapter. However, because you probably know a drug by its brand name, you can find information on it faster by checking out the alphabetical listing of brand names with their generic names at the end of this chapter. Use that generic name to find my discussion of a particular drug in the chapter.

Many of these drugs are available in combinations, which take advantage of the fact that two drugs of different classes are often more potent together than each one can be by itself. I list those many drug combinations by brand names at the end of their sections.

Diuretics

Of all the drug classes, the only one that has consistently reduced the illness and death associated with high blood pressure when it's the first treatment is the diuretic class, specifically the thiazide diuretics.

Diuretics, also known as *water pills,* lower blood pressure by forcing the body to rid itself of salt and water through the kidneys into the urine. They rid the body of more or less salt and water depending on where they're active in the kidneys (see Chapter 6 for details about the kidneys and their structure). After a couple of months, the body overcomes the reduction in body fluids. At this point, the reduction in the resistance to blood flow accounts for the ongoing fall in blood pressure. Diuretics are divided into different groups according to where they act along the *nephron* (the functional units in the kidney that remove waste and excess substances from the blood) as follows:

- **Thiazide and thiazidelike diuretic group:** Although they're *not* the most effective drugs for ridding the body of excess salt and water, this group *is* the most effective for lowering blood pressure. This group acts at the *distal tubule* (a part of the nephron where water and waste exchange occurs) to increase the excretion of sodium and chloride.

- **Loop diuretics:** This group acts at the thick ascending limb of the *loop of Henle,* part of the kidney's filtering mechanism. These drugs have a potent effect on salt and water elimination.

- **Potassium-sparing diuretics:** This group functions at the *late distal tubule* and the *collecting tubule* (key parts of the nephron's exchange system). The result is only a mild increase in sodium excretion and chloride excretion but a tendency to reduce the excretion of potassium. Because the other diuretics cause potassium loss, these potassium-sparing diuretics are important for maintaining body potassium.

- **Aldosterone-antagonist group:** This group blocks the action of *aldosterone,* a natural hormone that causes salt and water retention, so that more salt and water is excreted into the urine while potassium loss is reduced. These drugs could be included in the potassium-sparing group, but they lower blood pressure in an altogether different manner than the potassium-sparing group — they deactivate aldosterone.

Thiazide and thiazidelike diuretic group

Thiazide diuretics, the most effective blood-pressure-lowering drugs, have been prescribed for more than 40 years and have the following positive characteristics:

- Can be taken once daily (an important issue in patient compliance)

- Have low cost

- Are often as effective in low dosage as in higher dosage, thus reducing the side effects

- Lower the blood pressure about 15 mm Hg systolic and 7 mm Hg diastolic

- Appear to be better tolerated than other classes of drugs for high blood pressure because a lower percentage of people stop taking it

- Reduce the size of an enlarged heart (a sign of uncontrolled high blood pressure) about the same as the other classes of drugs

- Are especially useful among African Americans and the elderly

Common side effects of thiazide diuretics are as follows:

- ✔ Initially induce sleep loss due to urination (but this side effect is offset by taking medication early in the day)
- ✔ Reduce calcium excretion in the urine and may provoke elevated blood calcium levels
- ✔ Are not recommended during pregnancy and breast-feeding
- ✔ In higher dosage, cause excessive potassium loss, increase serum cholesterol, and increase the body's resistance to its own insulin (resulting in an increased intolerance to glucose, the sugar in the blood)

    Thiazides may increase a person's tendency toward diabetes.
- ✔ Causes problems with erection in men, especially in higher dosages
- ✔ Reduces the activity of certain drugs, especially insulin, *anticoagulants* (blood thinners), drugs to reduce uric acid in the blood, and *sulfonylureas* (antidiabetic drugs with names such as *chlorpropamide, tolazamide,* and *tolbutamide*)
- ✔ Increases the activity of vitamin D and certain drugs, particularly *digitalis* (a heart drug) and *lithium* (a drug for psychiatric impairment)

The following sections cover individual drugs within the thiazide and thiazidelike diuretic group.

Hydrochlorothiazide

Of all the thiazide diuretics, *hydrochlorothiazide* (HydroDIURIL, Hydrochlorothiazide Capsules, Hydrochlorothiazide Oral Solution, and Hydrochlorothiazide Tablets) is probably prescribed the most often. It has proven its value over many years and is effective in small doses. However, hydrochlorothiazide isn't recommended for people with kidney failure or an allergic hypersensitivity to drugs such as *sulfonamide* antibiotics. This diuretic must be used carefully when severe liver disease is present.

Some studies have shown that lower doses of hydrochlorothiazide actually reduce heart attacks more often than higher doses. If you're taking 50 mg or even more for high blood pressure, ask your doctor to lower the dose to 25 mg to see whether your blood pressure remains low. If so, try for 12.5 mg. The reduced frequency of side effects at this low dose makes such a trial worthwhile.

A 50-mg dose is associated with increased blood sugar and potassium loss, but a lower dose may make these side effects milder or disappear altogether. *Note:* If the blood glucose is extremely elevated, you may need to discontinue the drug. To counter the loss of potassium, a potassium-sparing agent may be combined with hydrochlorothiazide (oral potassium isn't nearly as effective, and it's hard to take). See more on these agents in the "Potassium-sparing diuretics" section later in this chapter.

The following symptoms suggest loss of too much potassium and body fluids:

- ✔ Confusion
- ✔ Drowsiness
- ✔ Dry mouth
- ✔ Muscle cramps and pains
- ✔ Nausea and vomiting
- ✔ Thirst
- ✔ Weakness

Call your doctor if several of these occur.

Hydrochlorothiazide comes in 25- and 50-mg pills. The recommended dosage is one 25-mg tablet daily, although starting with 12.5 mg daily, especially for an elderly person, is even better. Because the medication is eliminated from the body through the kidneys, it shouldn't be given when kidney failure is present.

Chlorothiazide

Chlorothiazide (Diuril Tablets, Diuril Oral Suspension, and Chlorothiazide Tablets) is almost identical to hydrochlorothiazide. All the information under hydrochlorothiazide also pertains to chlorothiazide.

Because of a slight difference in the chemical makeup, chlorothiazide has about one-tenth the potency of hydrochlorothiazide and comes in 250- and 500-mg tablets. The dose is 250 mg once or twice daily and more if the blood pressure is not controlled.

Bendroflumethiazide

Bendroflumethiazide (Naturetin) has a structure similar to hydrochlorothiazide and shares the same features (including the side effects), but it's ten times stronger than hydrochlorothiazide. This drug is being tested in the Hypertension in the Elderly Trial in Europe to see whether controlling the blood pressure in people age 80 and older causes a substantial reduction in brain attacks among that population.

Bendroflumethiazide has been used to suppress breast milk, which further verifies that it shouldn't be used during breast-feeding. It may also worsen *systemic lupus erythematosis* (commonly known as *lupus,* a chronic inflammatory disease in which immunological reactions cause abnormalities of blood vessels and connective tissue) if present.

Bendroflumethiazide comes as 5- and 10-mg tablets, and the dose is usually 2.5 to 5 mg daily or on alternate days. It's considerably more expensive than hydrochlorothiazide and chlorothiazide.

Hydroflumethiazide

In general, *Hydroflumethiazide* (Diucardin) has effects and side effects similar to those of hydrochlorothiazide. The kidneys excrete it, so it may accumulate in the presence of kidney disease. This med comes in 50-mg tablets. The starting dose is one tablet daily, and the maximum dose is 200 mg once daily. In high blood pressure treatment, 25 mg may be sufficient.

Methyclothiazide

Methyclothiazide (Methyclothiazide Tablets) is a variation of hydrochlorothiazide but it's ten times more potent than that drug. It's available as 2.5- or 5-mg tablets and has the same side effects as hydrochlorothiazide. The dosage is 2.5 mg once a day to start.

Chlorthalidone

Chlorthalidone (Thalitone, Chlorthalidone Tablets) differs chemically from hydrochlorothiazide and its effects tend to last longer, but its blood-pressure-lowering activity is about the same. The precautions associated with hydrochlorothiazide also pertain to chlorthalidone, which comes as 15-, 25-, 50- and 100-mg tablets. Only half the smallest tablet may be enough to control blood pressure. It's taken once daily.

Indapamide

Indapamide (Indapamide Tablets) is more like chlorthalidone than hydrochlorothiazide in its structure, but it has 20 times the potency of hydrochlorothiazide. Because it doesn't raise serum cholesterol, indapamide has an advantage over hydrochlorothiazide.

Indapamide is available at a dose of 1.5 or 2.5 mg with the usual once or twice daily treatment. However, a sustained-release preparation contains 1.5 mg that lasts throughout a 24-hour period with less effect on the potassium than the higher dosage. The 1.5-mg dosage is just as effective as 2.0 and 2.5 mg.

Metolazone

Metolazone (Mykrox, Zaroxolyn, Metolazone Tablets) is structurally different from hydrochlorothiazide but acts in much the same way. It's 20 times as potent. The advantage of Mykrox over Zaroxolyn and other diuretics is its rapid absorption and earlier activity. Although Zaroxolyn is the same drug, it's absorbed more slowly and isn't interchangeable with Mykrox.

Mykrox comes in 0.5-mg tablets. Zaroxolyn comes in 2.5-, 5-, and 10-mg dosages taken once a day. The precautions for both meds are the same as for hydrochlorothiazide.

Loop diuretics

Loop diuretics are more effective than the thiazide diuretics for ridding the body of salt and water, but they don't lower the blood pressure as much. Loop diuretics don't raise the cholesterol the way that thiazide diuretics do (a definite advantage), but they're not as effective in reducing disease and death caused by high blood pressure.

Loop diuretics reduce not only sodium and chloride but also calcium and magnesium. They're potent enough to cause a serious fall in the blood sodium if used to excess, and they can cause significant potassium loss. These dangers of loop diuretics make them less useful than thiazide diuretics (see the previous section) in the treatment of high blood pressure.

Other problems associated with the loop diuretics include

- Hearing loss or a ringing in the ears
- Serum uric acid increase with possible development of *gout,* a painful swelling of certain joints, especially the big toes
- Reactions in people who are hypersensitive to several sulphur-containing antibiotics and sulfonamides (this includes several drugs for treatment of diabetes like *diabinase* and *tolinase*).
- When mixed with the following medications, loop diuretics can cause problems:

  - **Anti-inflammatory agents:** Diminishes diuretic activity
  - **Blood thinners:** Tendency to bleed
  - **Digitalis:** Development of irregular heart rhythms
  - **Lithium:** Diarrhea and vomiting
  - **Probenecid:** Diminished diuretic activity
  - **Propranolol:** An exceptionally slow heart rate
  - **Sulfonylureas:** Low blood sugar

Chemically, loop diuretics are different from one another, unlike the drugs in the thiazide group. I describe the characteristics of some of the individual loop diuretics in the following sections.

The loop diuretics are dangerous when

- Kidneys have failed
- Sensitivity to the specific drug or to the sulfonamide class of drugs increases

Use during pregnancy and breast-feeding is probably not a good idea, but you can discuss this with your doctor.

Furosemide

Furosemide (Lasix, Furosemide Tablets, Furosemide Oral Solution) is the most commonly used member of the loop diuretics. Although it has a powerful effect on the expulsion of excess salt and water from the body, it can also cause excessive salt loss and dehydration. Furosemide also shares many of the problems associated with the thiazide diuretics. Among the most important are the following:

- ✔ Can't be taken if kidney failure or hypersensitivity to furosemide or sulfonamide drugs is present
- ✔ Must be taken carefully in the presence of severe liver disease
- ✔ Is not advisable for pregnant or breast-feeding women
- ✔ May result in dizziness on standing up when too much salt and water is lost
- ✔ Sensitizes skin to the sun
- ✔ Is associated with increased blood sugar
- ✔ Raises the blood uric acid (although rarely causes gout)
- ✔ Advances disease in someone with systemic lupus erythematosis

Furosemide also interacts with many other drugs. Depending on the frequency with which the other drugs are taken, the most important drug interactions include the following:

- ✔ Drugs already known to cause damage to hearing (like aspirin and some antibiotics) may cause even more damage.
- ✔ Lithium doesn't clear from the body as much as other drugs, and it may cause diarrhea and vomiting.
- ✔ Sucralfate (a drug used for treatment of stomach ulcers) may inhibit furosemide activity.

Checking the blood level of sodium, potassium, calcium, and magnesium frequently during the first few months of furosemide treatment is important. Ask your doctor whether your serum sodium and serum potassium are normal after a month of furosemide. If he can't give you an answer, ask to have these tests every six weeks or so for the first six months and then occasionally thereafter.

Furosemide comes in 20-, 40-, and 80-mg tablets. Most patients start by taking the lowest dose, which usually begins to work in about an hour and lasts for roughly eight hours, once each day. If necessary, a second dose can be taken during the day.

Ethacrynic acid

Ethacrynic acid (Edecrin Tablets) is similar in structure to furosemide but is slightly less potent. It shares the problems of this powerful group of diuretics and should probably not be used during pregnancy or breast-feeding.

Ethacrynic acid comes in 25- and 50-mg tablets taken one to three times a day as needed. For high blood pressure, 25 mg should be taken after a meal. It usually starts to work within 30 minutes and lasts for about eight hours.

Torsemide

Torsemide (Demadex) has three times the potency of furosemide. The liver does most of the metabolizing of this drug, so torsemide is particularly dangerous in the presence of severe liver disease.

Torsemide is available as 5-, 10-, 20-, and 100-mg tablets taken once a day. Patients can take it at any time (no need to consider meal times); it usually begins to work in an hour and lasts about eight hours. High blood pressure patients usually take the lowest dose for the first four to six weeks before the doctor reevaluates the dosage. Ten milligrams is usually the maximum dose for the treatment of high blood pressure.

Bumetanide

Bumetanide (Bumex, Bumetanide Tablets) is similar in structure and side effects to furosemide but is 40 times more potent. This drug has been associated with severe dehydration and loss of blood electrolytes like sodium and potassium. Older patients are especially at risk for severe dehydration. It hasn't been tested on children under age 18, so it's not recommended for this group.

Bumetanide is available as 0.5-, 1-, and 2-mg tablets. It usually begins to work in 30 to 60 minutes and lasts about six hours. Patients usually take it once a day in the morning, but if a single dose doesn't work long enough, your doctor may prescribe a second dose later in the day (before 6 p.m. to avoid waking up to urinate).

Potassium-sparing diuretics

Potassium-sparing diuretics have little effect on salt and water or lowering blood pressure, but in combination with other diuretics, they conserve the body's potassium. Therefore, they're often manufactured with a diuretic.

Their ability to conserve potassium is also their greatest danger — an abnormal elevation of the blood-potassium level — so they should never be used when the potassium is already high. People with diseases such as kidney failure are at a particularly high risk for this complication. These drugs also decrease the loss of calcium and magnesium associated with the other diuretics.

Amiloride

Amiloride (Midamor Tablets, Amiloride HCl Tablets) is used only with another diuretic to reverse the tendency of the other diuretic to excrete potassium in the urine. It also conserves magnesium.

Amiloride is eliminated almost equally by the kidneys and the liver; in the presence of kidney failure or liver disease, it can accumulate to dangerous, toxic levels.

Amiloride may also cause excessive potassium retention, so blood potassium levels must be monitored. (Muscle weakness, swelling of the abdomen, and diarrhea are symptomatic of excessive potassium retention.) Patients who have diabetes mellitus (see Chapter 4) are especially sensitive to the potassium-sparing effect of amiloride even when they don't have kidney disease. ***Note:*** Using salt substitutes and taking amiloride may put a patient at greater risk because salt substitutes contain *potassium* chloride instead of *sodium* chloride.

Amiloride isn't recommended during pregnancy or breast-feeding. It can decrease the excretion of lithium in the urine leading to lithium toxicity.

This drug comes in a 5-mg tablet, the usual dose. It starts to act in two hours and continues its activity for 24 hours.

Triamterene

Triamterene (Dyrenium) differs in structure from amiloride and has only one-tenth of amiloride's potency. It accomplishes the same task of conserving potassium in the patient taking a diuretic that causes potassium loss.

Because it leaves the body in the urine, triamterene shouldn't be taken when kidney failure or liver disease exists. Just like amiloride, it has to be monitored with frequent tests of blood potassium, especially in people with diabetes and the elderly (who are more likely to have high blood potassium levels). It's also not recommended during pregnancy and breast-feeding.

Triamterene comes as 50- and 100-mg tablets, usually starts to act in two to four hours, and lasts up to nine hours. As a result, patients usually need to take it twice a day, which is a disadvantage. It's taken after meals to avoid stomach upset.

Aldosterone-antagonist diuretics

Aldosterone-antagonist diuretics do not directly cause loss of salt and potassium in the urine. Instead, they block the action of the steroid hormone aldosterone (see Chapter 4), which causes salt and water retention. As a result, these diuretics cause salt and water loss only if aldosterone is present. At the same time, they conserve potassium, so these are also potassium-sparing drugs.

They must be used carefully when potassium is already elevated or when the patient is taking a drug that tends to raise potassium.

All the dangers of high potassium for the potassium-sparing diuretics (see the previous section) apply to aldosterone-antagonist diuretics.

Spironolactone

Spironolactone has a number of side effects because of its structure: breast enlargement in men and women, loss of potency, decreased interest in sex, increased hairiness, deepening of the voice, and menstrual irregularities. It can also cause sleepiness, confusion, headaches, and irritation and bleeding in the stomach.

The drug comes in 25-, 50-, and 100-mg tablets, usually starts to act only after one to two days, and continues to increase salt and urine output for two to three days. For high blood pressure, patients usually take 50 mg once a day along with a diuretic that causes potassium loss. Your doctor may be willing to reduce the dose to 25 mg with a good result.

Eplerenone

Eplerenone (Inspra) is a newer aldosterone antagonist with fewer side effects (particularly breast enlargement and sexual side effects) than spironolactone. It comes in 25- and 50-mg tablets. The dose starts at 50 mg and is given once or twice a day as needed. The potassium level is monitored on a weekly basis.

Diuretic combinations

If a patient takes a thiazide diuretic at the recommended low dosage, the possibility of excessive potassium loss is small (especially when the person eats a good diet), but it does occur. At higher doses, potassium loss is more likely. Because of the thiazide diuretics' tendency to cause potassium loss, drug companies have created a number of diuretic combinations. You may already be taking one or another of the combinations that follow (I have listed these by their brand names):

- **Amiloride Hydrochloride and Hydrochlorothiazide Tablets:** 5 mg amiloride plus 50 mg hydrochlorothiazide

- **Dyazide:** 37.5 mg triamterene and 25 mg hydrochlorothiazide

- **Maxide:** 75 mg Triamterene and 50 mg hydrochlorothiazide

- **Maxide-25:** 37.5 mg Triamterene and 25 mg hydrochlorothiazide

- **Moduretic:** 5 mg amiloride plus 50 mg hydrochlorothiazide

- **Triamterene and Hydrochlorothiazide Capsules and Tablets:** 37.5 mg triamterene and 25 mg hydrochlorothiazide

✔ **Triamterene and Hydrochlorothiazide Tablets:** 75 mg triamterene and 25 mg hydrochlorothiazide

✔ **Triamterene/HCTZ Capsules:** 50 mg triamterene and 25 mg hydrochlorothiazide

✔ **Triamterene/HCTZ Capsules and Tablets:** 37.5 mg triamterene and 25 mg hydrochlorothiazide

✔ **Triamterene/HCTZ Tablets:** 75 mg triamterene and 50 mg hydrochlorothiazide

✔ **Spironolactone and Hydrochlorothiazide Tablets:** 25 mg spironolactone and 25 mg hydrochlorothiazide

As you can see, numerous choices of tablets and capsules are available in a variety of amounts. Make sure you're getting the combination that your doctor wants you to have.

Drugs That Act on the Nervous System

The *sympathetic nervous system* is the part of the nervous system responsible for increased constriction of the arteries, thus raising blood pressure. This system uses hormones called *epinephrine* and *norepinephrine* to act as *neurotransmitters* (chemical messengers) along the nerves. When the brain wants action, like blood-vessel constriction, it sends out neurotransmitters that make the jump from the end of one nerve to the beginning of another nerve. Receptors located at the beginning of nerves take up the neurotransmitter so the signal can proceed down the nerve.

In 1940, researchers discovered that cutting the nerves of the sympathetic nervous system in the chest and abdomen caused a persistent fall in blood pressure. Since then, scientists have looked for chemical agents that could block the sympathetic nervous system, and they have come up with quite a bundle. These drugs lower blood pressure by affecting nerve transmission in the brain or outside the brain, and they're grouped by the *way* they affect the nervous system. In this section I explain each group in simple terms and then list the medications within each group.

Methyldopa

Methyldopa (Aldomet, Methyldopa Tablets; a drug that acts within the brain to prevent the release of neurotransmitters so they never get to the receptors) has a history of effectiveness and is still used by many physicians. It isn't usually the first drug of choice for high blood pressure because of the following rare but serious side effects:

✔ **Anemia:** Iron-deficient blood that causes red blood cell count to fall

✔ **Liver damage:** With fever and abnormal liver blood tests

Because of these side effects, patients should have blood count and liver tests before they start the drug and again every few months for the first year. If anemia or liver damage is discovered, the patient can stop taking the drug, which then usually eliminates these side effects.

Other side effects include

✔ **Decreased sex drive:** Some patients complain of this effect.

✔ **Dry mouth:** This may result from decreased saliva production.

✔ **Elevated levels of prolactin:** An elevated level of this brain hormone can cause an increase in breast size and formation of liquid in the breasts.

✔ **Sleepiness:** When methyldopa is first taken, the patient should be cautious about driving and running other complicated machinery.

Because the drug has been found safe for pregnant women, it's often the first choice for pregnant women with high blood pressure. It's found in breast milk, however, so it's not the best choice for a nursing mother.

Methyldopa comes in 125-, 250-, and 500-mg tablets. It usually begins to work in two hours, and its effect lasts about eight hours. Patients usually take a dose of 250 mg two or three times a day; the dosage is raised or lowered every few days until blood pressure control is achieved. The maximum dose is four 500-mg tablets a day. Methyldopa is eliminated from the body through the kidneys for the most part, so patients who have reduced kidney function require lower doses.

A combination of methyldopa and other drugs for high blood pressure, especially the thiazide diuretics, can be very effective. Various combinations include

✔ **Aldoclor:** 250 mg of methyldopa and 250 mg of chlorothiazide

✔ **Aldoril:** Methyldopa and hydrochlorothiazide in four strengths:

- **Aldoril-15:** 250 mg methyldopa and 15 mg hydrochlorothiazide
- **Aldoril-25:** 250 mg methyldopa and 25 mg hyrdrochlorothiazide
- **Aldoril-D30:** 500 mg methyldopa and 30 mg hydrochlorothiazide
- **Aldoril D50:** 500 mg methyldopa and 50 mg hydrochlorothiazide

✔ **Methyldopa and Hydrochlorothiazide Tablets** in two combinations:

- 250 mg methyldopa and 15 mg hydrochlorothiazide
- 250 mg methyldopa and 25 mg hydrochlorothiazide

Clonidine, guanabenz, and guanfacine

Clonidine, guanabenz, and *guanfacine* are similar drugs that lower blood pressure by reducing levels of norepinephrine. They reduce the output of blood from the heart and increase the size of arteries. Because of the sedation that they bring on (and the better characteristics of other drugs), they aren't the drug of choice for treating high blood pressure. These drugs are usually given with a diuretic.

These three drugs have similar side effects including

- **Sleepiness:** Best taken before bedtime; dosage increases occur at bedtime
- **Dry mouth:** May worsen to dry eyes and dryness of the nose
- **Disturbing dreams:** May cause depression and vivid dreams or nightmares

Discontinuation of these drugs, especially at higher doses, must be gradual because of withdrawal symptoms like headaches, shakiness, and a rise in arterial blood pressure *above* the original high level. Therefore, if you must quit taking it before surgery, your doctor will probably substitute another drug well in advance. (He may decide not to stop this drug at all, but you should be sure that you get it on the morning of your surgery.)

Clonidine

Clonidine (Catapres, Clonidine Hydrochloride Tablets, Clonidine HCl Tablets) comes in 0.1-, 0.2-, and 0.3-mg strengths. It's usually prescribed as a starting dose of 0.1 mg twice daily and changed on a weekly basis depending on the blood pressure. The maximum dose is usually 0.6 mg, although some doctors use more. It usually begins to act within an hour and lasts for roughly 12 hours.

- Clonidine is also marketed as Catapres-TTS, Catapres transdermal system, a patch containing 0.1, 0.2, or 0.3 mg that's applied to the skin. Each patch lasts a week — as long as it doesn't fall off.
- Clorpres is the brand name for a preparation that combines 0.1, 0.2, or 0.3 mg clonidine with 15 mg chlorthalidone.

Guanabenz

Guanabenz (Wytensin, Guanabenz Acetate Tablets) comes as 4- and 8-mg tablets. Patients usually start at 4 mg twice daily and increase to 8 mg twice daily. The maximum daily dose is 32 mg. Guanabenz usually begins to act in 1 hour and lasts about 12 hours. The dose may be changed every two weeks until the blood pressure is under control.

Guanfacine

Guanfacine (Tenex, Guanfacine Tablets, Guanfacine Hydrochloride Tablets) comes in 1- or 2-mg tablets. Patients usually start at 1 mg at bedtime. It begins to work in about two hours and lasts roughly 24 hours. The dosage can be changed every three to four weeks, up to a maximum dose of 3 mg daily.

Beta-adrenergic receptor blockers

Beta-adrenergic receptor blockers, generally known as *beta blockers,* are the most potent and side-effect-free group of drugs that affect the sympathetic nervous system and are second only to the thiazide diuretics in their effectiveness.

So many brand names are available that every drug manufacturer seems to have a version. And although they differ in certain respects, they all seem to have about the same effect on the blood pressure and are only slightly less effective than the diuretics. They're added to a patient's prescriptions when the thiazide diuretics don't completely control the blood pressure.

Beta blockers aren't the drug of first choice for high blood pressure unless the patient has a history of chest pain or heart attack. In these cases, beta blockers reduce the forcefulness of the heart while they reduce the secretion of renin and the production of angiotensin II (see Chapter 4). They also seem to protect patients with atherosclerotic heart disease (see Chapter 5) against pain and further disease.

Two different beta-adrenergic receptor blockers interrupt the sympathetic nervous system's activity: beta 1, which block beta-1 receptors; and beta 2, which block beta-2 receptors. ***Note:*** As the dose of the beta blocker rises, its specificity declines, and the same beta blocker blocks both receptors.

Beta blockers are especially useful for people with diseased blood vessels in the heart. This is particularly true of the beta-2 blockers like *propranolol* and *timolol,* which don't attach selectively to the nerves in the heart. Studies have shown that, unlike beta-1 blockers, these drugs are associated with a reduction in death rates. Choosing between propranolol and timolol comes down to cost because twice-daily propranolol is much less expensive than twice-daily timolol (if you use the nonbrand drug). But scientific evidence also indicates that propranolol is probably the best choice. If you want to make life a little easier (but more expensive), you can choose Inderal LA (brand name) for once-a-day dosing.

Beta blockers are associated with a number of side effects. The important ones are

- **Aggravated asthma:** They can make asthma worse.

- **Blocked heart:** Beta blockers can be harmful when the electrical conduction system of the heart is diseased.

- **Fatigue:** This effect may result from the decrease in blood flow to the brain when the blood pressure is lowered.

- **Heart attack:** Beta blockers have to be discontinued slowly to avoid precipitating heart pain and a heart attack.

- **Increased blood pressure if stopped:** If the patient suddenly stops taking these drugs, the blood pressure may rebound higher than the pretreatment level. These drugs should be lowered gradually over a couple of weeks.

- **Intolerance to exercise:** Beta blockers are not a good choice for the strenuous exerciser. They don't permit the heart to speed up for exercise.

- **Lower blood HDL:** Some of the beta blockers lower the blood HDL, the good cholesterol.

- **Lowered blood sugar:** Diabetics on these drugs may not respond properly to low blood sugar levels; the hormones that raise the blood sugar are dependent on the same nerves that beta blockers affect.

- **Retarded fetal growth:** Pregnant women should not use these drugs because they may retard the growth of the fetus.

- **Slower heart rate:** This effect contributes to the fatigue.

- **Toxicity:** In the presence of kidney failure or liver disease, beta blockers can accumulate because they're eliminated by the kidneys, the liver, or both.

Previously, researchers thought beta blockers were less effective for the elderly. This theory has been proven false, but beta blockers are known to be less effective among African Americans, particularly the diabetic population. The exception is *labetalol,* a drug that combines beta and alpha blockers (I discuss alpha blockers in the following section).

The characteristics of the various beta blockers (scientific names all end in *lol*) are as follows:

Acebutolol

Acebutolol (Sectral, Acebutolol Capsules, Acebutolol Hydrochloride Capsules) comes in 200-or 400-mg capsules. It's usually prescribed for once daily from 200 mg to a maximum of 1200 mg. The liver eliminates acebutolol more than the kidney does.

Atenolol

Atenolol (Tenormin, Atenolol Tablets) is available in 25-, 50-, or 100-mg tablets. The starting dose is usually 25 mg once a day up to a maximum of 200 mg once a day.

Atenolol also comes in combination form as Tenoretic 50 (50 mg of atenolol and 25 mg of the diuretic chlorthalidone) and Tenoretic 100 (100 mg of atenolol and 25 mg of chlorthalidone). Atenolol and Chlorthalidone Tablets are the same two combinations by another drug company. Atenolol in any form is eliminated by the kidney.

Bisoprolol

Bisoprolol (Zebeta) comes in 5- and 10-mg tablets. For high blood pressure, the starting dose is usually 5 mg, and some patients do well with half that dose. The maximum dose is 20 mg once a day. The characteristics of bisoprolol are similar to all other members of this group. Bisoprolol is eliminated by both the kidneys and the liver, so disease of either organ increases blood levels of the drug.

Carteolol

Carteolol (Cartrol Filmtab Tablets) comes in 2.5- or 5-mg tablets. Usually 2.5 mg is taken once a day up to a maximum of 10 mg once daily. This drug is eliminated more by the kidney than the liver.

Carvedilol

Carvedilol (Coreg) comes as 3.125-, 6.25-, 12.5-, and 25-mg tablets. The starting dose is usually 6.25 mg twice daily up to a maximum daily amount of 50 mg divided into two doses. The liver breaks down carvedilol, so people with liver disease may accumulate this drug in their bloodstream.

Labetalol

Labetalol (Trandate, Labetalol HCl Tablets) comes as 100-, 200-, and 300-mg tablets. It differs from most of the other beta blockers because of its effect on *alpha receptors* (see the following section), which then often causes dizziness. The drug has been associated with fever and liver abnormalities. The dose is usually 100 mg twice daily up to 1200 mg divided into two doses. The liver is the major organ of elimination.

Metoprolol

Metoprolol (Lopressor, Metoprolol Tartrate Tablets) comes in 50- and 100-mg strengths. The usual dose is 50 mg twice a day up to a daily maximum of 200 mg.

A slow-release form of this drug, Toprol XL, is usually prescribed for once a day. It comes in 25-, 50-, 100-, and 200-mg tablets. Elimination of both metoprolol and Toprol XL is by the liver.

Nadolol

Nadolol (Corgard, Nadolol Tablets) comes in 20-, 40-, 80-, 120-, and 160-mg tablets. The starting dose is usually 20 mg once daily up to 160 mg once daily. The kidney is the main site of elimination.

Nadolol also comes in combination with a thiazide diuretic (bendroflumethiazide) called Corzide. The tablets are either 40 mg of nadolol with 5 mg of bendroflumethiazide or 80 mg of nadolol with 5 mg of bendroflumethiazide.

Penbutolol

Penbutolol (Levatol) comes as a 20-mg tablet. The dose is usually 20 mg once a day up to 80 mg once a day. The kidneys eliminate penbutolol more than the liver.

Pindolol

Pindolol (Pindolol Tablets) comes in 5- and 10-mg strengths. The dose is usually 5 mg twice daily up to a maximum of 60 mg divided into two doses. The liver eliminates more of this drug than the kidneys.

Propranolol

Propranolol (Inderal Tablets, Propranolol Hydrochloride Oral Solution, Propranolol Hydrochloride Tablets) comes in 10-, 20-, 40-, 60-, and 80-mg strengths. The initial prescription is usually 20 mg twice daily up to 320 mg divided into two doses. This drug was the earliest of the beta blockers, so doctors have the most experience with it. It's eliminated by the liver.

Propranolol has a long-acting form called Inderal LA (60-, 80-, 120-, or 160-mg strengths) and InnoPran XL (80- and 120-mg extended-release form), which allows for once-a-day dosing. It also comes in combination with hydrochlorothiazide called Inderide or Propranolol Hydrochloride in two different strengths, 40 or 80 mg of propranolol plus 25 mg hydrochlorothiazide. Finally, a long-acting preparation of Inderide (Inderide LA) contains 80, 120, or 160 mg of propranolol plus 50 mg hydrochlorothiazide; it can be taken once a day.

Timolol

Timolol (Blocadren, Timolol Maleate Tablets) comes as 5-, 10-, or 20-mg tablets. The dose is usually 5 mg twice daily up to 40 mg divided into two doses. Timolol is eliminated by the liver more than the kidneys.

Timolol is also manufactured in combination with hydrochlorothiazide as Timolide 10-25 consisting of 10 mg of timolol and 25 mg of the diuretic. It also comes in solutions for the eye that lower elevated pressure in the eye.

Alpha-1 adrenergic receptor antagonists

Alpha-1 adrenergic receptor antagonists (alpha blockers) block another group of sympathetic nerve receptors, some of which are alpha 1 (located in smooth, muscle-like blood vessels) and some of which are alpha 2 (located where nerves connect to each other). Only the alpha-1 blockers are used clinically because they relax muscles in blood vessels to increase the size of the vessel and lower the blood pressure. They also lower the bad fats (triglycerides and LDL cholesterol) and raise the good fat (HDL cholesterol). The changes are small, however, and they can be associated with dizziness on standing.

Some unwanted side effects of these drugs include

- ✔ Increased occurrence of heart failure

  This tendency means the drug should be combined with a diuretic; it shouldn't be taken alone.

- ✔ *First-dose phenomenon* (the blood pressure drops very low after the first dose or when the drug dose is rapidly increased)

  This effect is especially common for patients already on a diuretic or a beta blocker. The patient should avoid driving or difficult tasks for the first 24 hours after the first dose, which should be taken at bedtime. The effect goes away after the first few doses.

- ✔ Tendency to lose their potency when the body gets used to them

The various drugs in this group include the following:

Doxazosin

Doxazosin (Cardura, Doxazosin) comes in 1-, 2-, 4-, and 8-mg tablets with a starting dose of 1 mg at bedtime that can go up to 16 mg once a day. ***Note:*** Doxazosin is not a good choice for a pregnant or nursing woman. Dizziness and fatigue occur in many of the patients who take it. It's eliminated by the liver.

A longer-acting preparation (Cardura XL) comes in 4- and 8-mg tablets. Both forms have been used in benign prostatic hypertrophy (non-cancerous enlargement of the prostate) as well as in high blood pressure.

Prazosin

Prazosin (Minipress, Prazosin HCl Capsules, Prazosin Hydrochloride Capsules, Prazosin HCl Capsules) comes as 1-, 2-, and 5-mg tablets. It's usually taken at a starting dose of 1 mg at bedtime up to 20 mg daily in two or three divided doses. Prazosin isn't recommended for women who are pregnant or breast-feeding. It's eliminated by the liver.

Terazosin

Terazosin (Hytrin, Terazosin Capsules, Terazosin Hydrochloride Capsules, Terazosin Tablets) is produced in 1-, 2-, 5-, and 10-mg strengths. The initial daily dose is 1 mg at bedtime rising to 20 mg divided into two doses if necessary. It also may reduce the size of the prostate gland in men. The liver eliminates terazosin.

Because of their tendency to cause side effects, these drugs have become less popular. They should be used with a thiazide diuretic.

Vasodilators

Vasodilators are drugs that relax the muscles in the arteries, making them larger and reducing blood pressure. How this occurs is unclear. When taken alone, these drugs cause

- The heart to speed up as the blood pressure falls
- The patient to suffer from headaches
- The feeling of a rapid heart beat
- Retention of water

Therefore, vasodilators are usually taken with diuretics (to get rid of water) and beta blockers (to slow the heart). Doctors usually reserve the use of two vasodilators, *hydralazine* and *minoxidil,* for the most difficult cases because of their side effects.

Hydralazine

Although *hydralazine* (Apresoline, Hydralazine HCl Tablets) was one of the earliest drugs for high blood pressure, it was seldom prescribed because it caused rapid heart beat and lost its effectiveness after a patient took it for a while (the body compensated for the open blood vessels by increasing heart rate and retaining water). Now that doctors understand it, they can prescribe other drugs to counteract this compensation and, as a result, restore hydralazine's effectiveness.

Hydralazine is rarely used in elderly patients because of the side effects. It has been prescribed for pregnant women and has been useful for severe high blood pressure during pregnancy. However, it shouldn't be prescribed to a nursing mother.

Because the drug is broken down mostly in the liver and then eliminated by the kidneys, anyone with liver or kidney disease must take this drug with care. When taken alone, hydralazine also causes retention of water and can result in heart failure (another reason for the addition of a diuretic and a beta blocker).

Hydralazine's other side effects include headaches, nausea, excess reduction in blood pressure, feeling of a rapid heartbeat, dizziness, and heart pain if there is coronary artery disease. Interestingly, although hydralazine expands some arteries of the heart, it doesn't expand certain other arteries in the heart. The result is that blood is stolen from one area by another, and the area that loses blood may develop pain.

Hydralazine can also cause an allergic reaction *(lupus syndrome)* against the body's own tissues after six months of treatment (and more frequently as the dose goes higher). *Slow acetylators* (patients who break down the drug slowly) get this condition more often than *fast acetylators*. The symptoms consist of fever, rash, itching, pain in the joints, and actual swelling, redness, and heat in the joints. After the drug is stopped, the condition usually subsides.

Hydralazine is available in 10-, 25-, 50-, and 100-mg strengths. It's usually taken twice daily; its action lasts about 12 hours. The maximum dose is 200 mg divided into two doses. Because it's not active after the liver breaks it down, fast acetylators (about 50 percent of the patients) need higher doses of the drug than slow acetylators.

Hydralazine is also available in combination form as Hydra-Zide Capsules, a combination of hydralazine and hydrochlorothiazide in the following proportions:

- 25 mg hydralazine and 25 mg hydrochlorothiazide
- 50 mg hydralazine and 50 mg hydrochlorothiazide
- 100 mg hydralazine and 50 mg hydrochlorothiazide

Minoxidil

Minoxidil (Loniten, Minoxidil Tablets) was discovered in 1965 and controls the most severe and resistant cases of high blood pressure. It relaxes *smooth muscle* (the muscle in the walls of arteries) and is most useful for severe high blood pressure that doesn't respond to other agents. It's always administered with a diuretic and a beta blocker to reverse its undesirable side effects.

The drug is broken down in the liver and then eliminated by the kidneys, so disease of either of these organs causes minoxidil to accumulate in the body. Minoxidil has been used in children, but it's not recommended for pregnant women or women who are breast-feeding. The following side effects complicate the use of this powerful drug:

- ✔ Salt and water retention because the pressure in the kidney's nephrons (see Chapter 6 for details about nephrons) is reduced

  Taking a diuretic along with the minoxidil reverses this effect.

- ✔ Increased heart rate along with the strength of heart contractions

  If coronary artery disease already exists (see Chapter 5 for more info), heart pain can result from the increased work of the heart. A beta-blocking drug can control this side effect. If the heart has been close to failure, minoxidil may worsen the problem so that heart failure occurs.

- ✔ Increased hair growth on the face, back, arms, and legs after a person is on the drug for several months

  This is a problem for women especially. Minoxidil is now used commercially in the form of Rogaine for treatment of baldness.

Minoxidil is available in 2.5- and 10-mg tablets. The starting dose may be as little as 1.25 mg once daily up to a maximum of 40 mg once daily, and it begins to work in about 30 minutes.

Calcium Channel Blocking Agents

Calcium channel blocking agents (also known as *calcium channel blockers*) take advantage of the fact that calcium has to move into the muscle cell in order for a muscle in an artery to contract. These agents block that movement so the muscle can then relax. The result is larger arteries and lower blood pressure. Therefore, they act like a vasodilator but the mechanism is different.

As arteries widen and peripheral resistance declines, the body responds by increasing the heart rate. This result isn't true of all calcium channel blocking agents; certain calcium channel blocking agents, particularly *verapamil* and *diltiazem,* slow the heart so the heart rate doesn't increase.

For people with enlarged hearts or heart failure, calcium channel blockers aren't the first or second drug of choice for blood pressure treatment. Calcium channel blockers also shouldn't be the first or second choice of treatment for high blood pressure after a heart attack. They decrease muscle contraction — an undesirable effect when the heart is already failing or weakened by a heart attack.

Note: When heart disease doesn't already exist, calcium channel blockers can lower blood pressure as effectively as beta blockers. However, when a heart attack has occurred, calcium channel blockers don't improve survival as well as beta blockers.

Calcium channel blockers have several side effects, but these effects rarely cause the patient to stop taking the drug. The main side effects are headache, flushing in the face, dizziness, and swelling of the legs. To overcome these side effects, sustained-release preparations have been developed. However, these preparations don't help the swelling.

Another side effect that may make the patient uncomfortable is irritation of the *esophagus* (the passageway from the mouth to the stomach) and the stomach; the drugs slow down the passage of food from the stomach to the intestine. Constipation is also common with some of the agents in this class, (verapamil, diltiazem, and *nifedipine*).

Calcium channel blockers are effective in most patients when the preceding problems are taken into account. They work especially well in *low-renin* high blood pressure (most frequent among the elderly and African Americans). Of course, heart failure and heart attacks are also most frequent in the elderly, so this factor is a consideration.

Interactions with other drugs are important. The metabolism of *digoxin,* an important drug for the heart, is blocked, so digoxin can accumulate to toxic levels, resulting in severe abnormal heart rhythms.

Because calcium channel blockers are safe in the presence of diabetes, asthma, kidney abnormalities, and abnormal levels of blood fats, these drugs can be useful even though they're not the first choice for treating high blood pressure.

A number of calcium channel blockers are available. They're classified by their chemical structures:

- ✔ Underlying chemical structures are not similar *(verapamil and diltiazem).*

- ✔ Underlying chemical structures are similar *(amlodipine, felodipine, asradipine, nicardipine, nifedipine,* and *nisoldipine)* and end in *pine.*

Given all the choices in the following sections, which of these is the best for you? Keep in mind that a calcium channel blocker isn't the drug of choice for treating high blood pressure. If a combination of a diuretic and a beta blocker isn't sufficient, then calcium channel blockers may be considered.

The second group of drugs (beginning with amlodipine) is slightly more effective, although diltiazem and verapamil have fewer side effects. Little difference exists among the second group, so you may want to choose the least expensive extended-release tablet, Nifedipine Extended-release Tablets. Naturally, your doctor makes the decision, but you can influence her if you come prepared with the information in this chapter.

Verapamil and diltiazem

Verapamil (Calan, Covera, Isoptin, Verelan, Verapamil HCl Tablets, Verapamil Hydrochloride Tablets) is available in tablets containing 40, 80, and 120 mg of the drug. The dose is usually 80 mg three times a day up to 360 mg divided into three doses. Most of the drug is excreted into the urine, but about 20 percent leaves in the bowel movement. When liver or kidney disease is present, the drug may accumulate.

Long-acting preparations of verapamil are available:

- **Calan SR** containing 120, 180, or 240 mg may be taken once a day with food.
- **Covera-HS** is available as 180 and 240 mg tablets taken at bedtime.
- **Isoptin SR** is identical to Calan SR.
- **Verelan** is a sustained-release capsule available in strengths of 120, 180, 240, and 360 mg and may be taken once in the morning.
- **Verelan PM** is a capsule containing 100, 200, or 300 mg of verapamil and is taken at bedtime.
- **Verapamil Hydrochloride Extended-release Capsules and Tablets** are similar to Calan SR.

Diltiazem (Cardizem, Cardizem CD Capsules, Cartia XT, Tiazac, Taztia XT, Dilacor XR, Dilt CD, Diltia XT, Diltiazem Extended Release Capsules, Diltiazem Hydrochloride Extended Release Capsules, Diltaizem Hydrochloride Tablets) is usually sold in the extended-release form for once-a-day dosing. The liver processes diltiazem, so toxicity is likely to occur in the presence of liver disease. *Note:* Decreased kidney function doesn't seem to affect it. The side effects of diltiazem are just like those of verapamil, but it's less likely to cause constipation and more likely to cause heart failure.

It comes in 120-, 180-, 240-, 300-, and 360-mg capsules and tablets. The starting dose is usually 180 mg daily up to a maximum of 360 mg once daily.

Other calcium channel blockers

The drugs in the previous section are the more common calcium channel blockers. Their structures differ from each other and from the following drugs, which have similar structures:

- *Amlodipine* (Norvasc) doesn't often interact with other drugs, but it isn't recommended during pregnancy or when breast-feeding. It doesn't have severe side effects, and few patients have to stop the drug because of them. A small number of men complain of impotency with this drug.

Amlodipine is broken down in the liver, and the breakdown products are eliminated in the urine. Liver disease causes amlodipine to accumulate, but kidney disease doesn't affect the dosing.

This drug comes in 2.5-, 5-, and 10-mg tablets. Its initial prescription is usually 5 mg once daily with a maximum of 10 mg once a day. Elderly people usually start at 2.5 mg. It is sold in combination with benazepril as Lotrel in many different strengths (I discuss benazepril in more detail in the next section).

✔ *Felodipine* (Plendil) has the same side effects and elimination as amlodipine and the same precautions for pregnant and nursing women. It comes as an extended-release tablet in 2.5-, 5-, and 10-mg strengths. The starting dose is usually 5 mg, and the maximum is 10 mg once a day. It's taken without food or with a light meal and swallowed whole. Felodipine also comes in combination with enalapril (see more on this in the next section) in a product called Lexxel, which is manufactured as 5 mg of enalapril and 5 mg of felodipine.

✔ *Nicardipine* (Cardene, Nicardipine Capsules, Nicardipine Hydrochloride) shares all the characteristics of amlodipine and comes as 20- and 30-mg capsules. The starting dose is usually 20 mg three times daily and the maximum dose is 120 mg divided in three doses. This three-times-a-day dosing is a definite disadvantage when compared to the others of this group. A slow release form (Cardene SR) contains 30, 45, or 60 mg.

✔ *Nifedipine* (Adalat Capsules, Procardia Capsules) has the same side effects as amlodipine. It is available as 10- or 20-mg capsules. The dose is usually 10 mg three times daily up to 120 mg divided into three doses. Because of the inconvenience of three daily doses, extended-release formulations (Adalat CC Extended Release Tablets, Procardia XL Extended Release Tablets, and Nifedipine Extended-release Tablets) are available. These come in strengths of 30, 60, and 90 mg.

✔ *Nisoldipine* (Sular) shouldn't be taken with a high-fat meal, which leads to excessive release and a high concentration. Otherwise, the description of nisoldipine doesn't differ from amlodipine. It is an extended-release tablet available in strengths of 10, 20, 30, and 40 mg. The starting dose is usually 20 mg once a day up to a maximum of 60 mg once a day.

Angiotensin-Converting Enzyme Inhibitors

Angiotensin-converting enzyme (ACE) *inhibitors* affect the activity of the renin-angiotensin-aldosterone system (see Chapter 4). The body's angiotensin-converting enzyme converts a hormone (angiotensin I) to angiotensin II, which raises blood pressure two ways: It causes direct contraction of arteries; and it causes the adrenal gland to release aldosterone, which, in turn, causes salt and water retention. The ACE inhibitors block the enzyme to prevent the production of angiotensin II. ACE inhibitors can make thiazide diuretics more effective by blocking the body's tendency to make more aldosterone as it loses water and salt.

In addition to preventing the *increase* in blood pressure, the ACE inhibitor also leads to a *fall* in blood pressure. (Angiotensin II breaks down *bradykinen,* a hormone that causes widening of blood vessels. Without angiotensin II, bradykinen levels increase.)

This class of drugs is especially important and useful for people with heart failure, kidney disease, diabetes, and other kidney problems. More than any other drug for high blood pressure, ACE inhibitors slow the progression of these diseases.

ACE inhibitors have two major advantages:

- ✔ They don't cause a fall in potassium or changes in blood fats, blood sugar, or uric acid.
- ✔ They have a low number of side effects.

However, their potential side effects include the following:

- ✔ May lead to elevations in serum potassium levels (especially in patients with heart failure, diabetes, or reduced kidney function) by blocking aldosterone production
- ✔ May lead to abnormally low blood pressure if the patient already has decreased blood volume (for example, after treatment with a diuretic)
- ✔ May cause a dry cough (20-percent chance), which can be very annoying.
- ✔ Rarely lead to a rash, loss of taste, and reduction of white blood cells
- ✔ A very rare but potentially fatal complication is *angioneurotic edema,* which causes the throat to swell severely so breathing becomes very difficult. These drugs should be stopped immediately if such signs and symptoms develop.

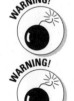

An ACE inhibitor should not be

- ✔ Paired with a potassium-sparing diuretic or spironolactone; the combination can be dangerous because both meds cause increased blood potassium.
- ✔ Used during pregnancy or in a young woman who plans to become pregnant soon because ACE inhibitors can damage the growing fetus.
- ✔ Used during breast-feeding (to avoid damage to the nursing infant).

These drugs aren't as effective among African Americans unless given with a diuretic (probably because this high blood pressure isn't normally driven by angiotensin II). However, elderly people with angiotensin-II-driven high blood pressure do respond just like younger people to ACE inhibitors.

Compared to diuretics, beta blockers, and calcium channel blockers, ACE inhibitors don't lower blood pressure as effectively. In terms of decreasing sickness and death, ACE inhibitors are less effective than diuretics and beta blockers but more effective than calcium channel blockers.

Numerous ACE inhibitors are available, and they have some variations in their breakdown. You can recognize them by the *pril* at the end of their names. Their characteristics are as follows:

- *Benazepril* (Lotensin), available as 5-, 10-, 20-, and 40-mg tablets, is usually prescribed initially at a dose of 10 mg daily and, if needed, rising to 40 mg once a day or in two doses.

  Patients who are already on a diuretic and then start benazepril are at risk for very low blood pressure. The recommendation is to stop the diuretic for several days first and add it back *if* the ACE inhibitor doesn't control the blood pressure. Alternately, the starting dose of benazepril can be lowered to 5 mg. Because the kidneys eliminate this drug in part, patients with severe kidney function loss need to take reduced doses.

  Benazepril is also available in combination with hydrochlorothiazide (Lotensin HCT). The proportions are benazepril 5 mg, hydrochlorothiazide 6.25 mg; 10 mg/12.5 mg; 20 mg/12.5 mg; and 20 mg/25 mg. Benazepril is also packaged with the calcium channel blocker amlodipine as Lotrel. The proportions are 2.5 mg amlodipine and 10 mg benazepril; 5 mg/ 10 mg; and 5 mg/20 mg.

- *Captopril* (Capoten, Captopril Tablets) was the first ACE inhibitor. It comes in 12.5-, 25-, 50-, and 100-mg strengths and is usually started at 25 mg twice daily; it can be increased up to 150 mg daily in two or three doses. Because food decreases the uptake of this drug, it should be taken an hour before meals. Most of the drug is eliminated in the urine, so people with decreased kidney function take less. Captopril seems to cause skin rashes and problems with taste more than the other ACE inhibitors. *Note:* The precaution for patients on a diuretic and benazepril (see the first bullet) applies to captopril and all the other ACE inhibitors.

  Captopril is also sold in a combination with hydrochlorothiazide as Captopril and Hydrochlorothiazide Tablets. The proportions are captopril 25 mg, hydrochlorothiazide 15 mg; 50 mg/15 mg; 25 mg/25 mg; and 50 mg/25 mg.

- *Enalapril* (Vasotec) comes in 2.5-, 5-, 10-, and 20-mg tablets. The usual dose is 5 mg once a day rising to 40 mg once a day or divided into two doses. The kidneys eliminate it, so less is taken in the presence of diminished kidney function.

  Vaseretic is a combination of enalapril and hydrochlorothiazide in the following proportions: 5 mg/12.5 mg and 10 mg/25 mg. Lexxel is a combination of enalapril and felodipine (see the earlier section on felodipine).

✔ *Fosinopril* (Monopril), available as 10-, 20-, and 40-mg tablets, is usually started at 10 mg once a day rising to 80 mg at most. If the blood pressure isn't low enough at the end of the single-dose period, the patient may divide the dose into two times a day. Because Fosinopril is broken down in the liver, the usual dose can be given even when severe kidney disease is present.

✔ *Lisinopril* (Prinivil, Zestril) comes in many strengths: 2.5, 5, 10, 20, 30, and 40 mg. The starting dose is from 10 to 40 mg once a day. The kidneys eliminate Lisinopril from the body, so the dose should be reduced if kidney function is poor.

Lisinopril also comes with hydrochlorothiazide as Zestoretic. It contains 10 mg of lisinopril and 12.5 mg of the diuretic; 20 mg/12.5 mg; or 20 mg/ 25 mg. Prinzide contains the same two drugs in the same proportions.

✔ *Moexipril* (Univasc) is available as 7.5- and 15-mg tablets. The dose usually starts at 7.5 mg once a day at least an hour before a meal. The maximum dose is 30 mg, which can be divided. Both liver disease and kidney disease prolong the activity of moexipril, so the dose should be reduced in both cases. Uniretic is a combination of moexipril and hydrochlorothiazide in the following proportions: 7.5 mg/12 mg and 15 mg/25 mg.

✔ *Perindopril* (Aceon), available in 2-, 4-, and 8-mg tablets, is usually started at 4 mg up to a maximum of 16 mg once a day. Doses should be reduced in the presence of decreased kidney function.

✔ *Quinapril* (Accupril) is supplied as 5-, 10-, 20-, and 40-mg tablets. The starting dose is usually 10 mg a day, and the maximum is 80 mg once a day or divided. *Note:* This drug doesn't reach its usual blood levels when taken with a high-fat meal. Because it's eliminated by the kidneys, the dose should be reduced if kidney failure is present.

Accuretic is a combination of quinapril and hydrochlorothiazide. The proportions are quinapril 10 mg and hydrochlorothiazide 12.5 mg; 20 mg/12.5 mg; and 20 mg/25 mg.

✔ *Ramipril* (Altace) is made in 1.25-, 2.5-, 5-, and 10-mg capsules. The dose is usually 2.5 mg to start, and the maximum dose is 20 mg once daily or divided into two doses. Dosage should be lowered in the presence of kidney disease.

✔ *Trandolapril* (Mavik) comes as 1-, 2-, and 4-mg tablets. The initial dose is usually 1 mg once daily adjusted up to 4 mg once daily. Dosage should be reduced in the presence of severe disease of the liver or kidneys.

Tarka is trandolapril and the calcium channel blocker verapamil. The proportions are 2 mg and 180 mg; 1 mg/240 mg; 2 mg/240 mg; and 4 mg/ 240 mg.

Why, you may ask, are all these different ACE inhibitors necessary? I don't know. ACE inhibitors aren't the drug of choice for high blood pressure but may be used when the diuretics or beta blockers can't be used. ACE inhibitors are particularly useful in the presence of heart failure or diabetic kidney disease. They're unique because they're free of most side effects.

How do you choose a particular ACE inhibitor? That question's a little easier to answer. A once-a-day drug is probably better, although most of them need to be taken twice a day when the dose is raised. Your insurance company will probably dictate which one you use because it's paying the bill (which also makes the decision fairly easy). But if you have to pay for it directly, I suggest you choose the cheapest drug.

Angiotensin II Receptor Blockers

Unlike ACE inhibitors (which block the angiotension-converting enzyme), an *angiotensin II receptor blocker* doesn't allow an enzyme to attach to its receptor where the receptor contracts arteries and releases aldosterone. These blockers are necessary because ACE inhibitors aren't effective against other enzymes that make angiotensin II. These receptor blockers, then, can eliminate the activity of angiotensin II more completely. Drugs in this group all end with *artan*.

Like the ACE inhibitors, these drugs are similar to one another. Advantages of Angiotensin II Receptor Blockers include the following:

- ✔ Effectively reverse kidney disease in diabetes even when the drugs *(irbesartan and losartan)* don't lower the blood pressure much

- ✔ Are relatively free of side effects, although they can elevate potassium (their action is similar to the ACE inhibitors')

- ✔ Are metabolized in the body into inactive substances, so elimination doesn't depend on the liver or the kidneys

- ✔ Don't change blood-fat levels, increase the uric acid, or increase the sugar in the blood

- ✔ Don't cause a dry cough like ACE inhibitors do

Occasional patients (less than 1 percent of those who take these drugs) develop headache or dizziness and have to discontinue the drugs. A rare patient develops facial swelling. Drug interactions don't seem to be a problem with this class.

Like the ACE inhibitors, Angiotensin II receptor blockers shouldn't be prescribed for pregnant or breast-feeding women or women who plan to become pregnant soon.

The various drugs and their properties are as follows:

- ✔ *Candesartan* (Atacand) comes as 4-, 8-, 16-, and 32-mg tablets. The usual starting dose is 16 mg up to a maximum of 32 mg once a day. The dose does not need to be adjusted for mild liver or kidney disease. Atacand-HCT is a combination of 16 or 32 mg of candesartan plus 12.5 mg of hydrochlorothiazide.

- ✔ *Eprosartan* (Teveten) is available as 400- and 600-mg tablets. Starting at 400 mg once daily, the maximum dose is 800 mg once daily. The dose doesn't have to be adjusted for kidney disease or liver disease.

- ✔ *Irbesartan* (Avapro) is manufactured as 75-, 150-, and 300-mg tablets. Starting at 150 mg once a day, the dose can go up to 300 mg once a day.

  Avalide is a combination of irbesartan and hydrochlorothiazide. The proportions are 150 or 300 mg of irbesartan with 12.5 or 25 mg of hydrochlorothiazide.

- ✔ *Losartan* (Cozaar) was the first member of this class to be approved by the FDA. It comes as 25-, 50-, and 100-mg tablets. Treatment usually begins with 50 mg and goes up to 100 mg as a single dose or divided in half and taken twice a day.

  Hyzaar is losartan with hydrochlorothiazide. The dose is usually 50 mg losartan and 12.5 mg of the diuretic or 100 mg losartan and 12.5 or 25 mg of the diuretic.

- ✔ *Olmesartan* (Benicar) comes in 5-, 20-, and 40-mg tablets. It is given at a starting dose of 20 mg to a maximum dose of 40 mg once daily.

- ✔ *Telmisartan* (Miscardis) is made in 20-, 40-, and 80-mg tablets. The beginning dose is usually 40 mg once a day up to 80 mg once a day. Miscardis HCT is a combination of telmisartan and hydrochlorothiazide with 40 or 80 mg of telmisartan and 12.5 or 25 mg of the diuretic.

- ✔ *Valsartan* (Diovan) is produced in 40-, 80-, 160-, and 320-mg capsules. Starting with 80 mg, the dose can go up to 320 mg once a day.

  Diovan HCT is valsartan plus hydrochlorothiazide. The proportions are 80, 160, or 320 mg of valsartan plus 12.5 or 25 mg of hydrochlorothiazide.

Quick, make your selection before you have 12 other copies of the same drug to confuse you! But keep this in mind: Angiotensin II receptor blockers are not the first choice for high blood pressure therapy because they don't lower blood pressure to the same extent. If possible, ask your doctor to prescribe one of the drugs that's the least expensive and that can be taken once a day.

Note: The angiotensin II receptor blockers are about twice as expensive as the ACE inhibitors. But are they twice as good? It doesn't appear so. Nevertheless, the angiotensin II receptor blockers may be a good solution for the person who cannot tolerate the cough caused by ACE inhibitors.

Choosing a Drug

Now that you know all about the drugs to control blood pressure, you're ready to put that information to use. Sure, your doctor makes the decisions about which medication to use, but you have the right to have some input because that drug goes into *your* body, not your doctor's. Unfortunately, as brilliant as doctors are, sometimes they base decisions on faulty information. Of course, it's never anything as obvious as which drug company representative is most alluring, but it may be a matter of which drug the doctor hears about most often. These medical decisions should always be based on evidence that a given drug is the best one for the situation.

Treating uncomplicated high blood pressure

Basic principles for starting treatment include the following:

1. **Ideally, use a drug that's cheap, has few side effects, and can be taken once a day.**

2. **Start with a very low dose, maybe half the recommended dose;** this is especially important for the elderly because they take many other drugs and have other diagnoses like heart failure, kidney disease, and liver disease.

3. **Increase the dose slowly until the desired effect is reached.**

4. **Add a second drug with a different mechanism of action if the pressure isn't controlled at a reasonable dose.** Again, start at a low dose and build up gradually.

5. **Discontinue it and try a drug with a different mechanism of action if you can't tolerate the drug because of side effects.**

6. **Always make sure your prescription is for enough medication to last until the next appointment and that you have a return appointment before leaving the office.**

7. **Improve your patient compliance by understanding the necessity for the drug, the exact treatment plan, and possible side effects — hence this book.** The largest barrier to good treatment is lack of patient compliance.

These principles assume that you don't have heart failure, eye disease, kidney disease, heart attacks, or other complications. Basically, you've lost weight, started an exercise program, reduced your dietary salt, and tried one or several of the alternative treatments in Chapter 12, but your doctor says your blood pressure is still too high on several occasions and it needs to be treated.

Take the following steps:

1. **Start with a diuretic, preferably hydrochlorothiazide, at a low dose of 12.5 or 25 mg daily.**

   Give this at least two months to lower your blood pressure while you get your potassium checked every few weeks.

2. **If the potassium falls abnormally low, add a potassium-sparing agent, probably amiloride.**

3. **Add a beta-blocking drug if necessary because higher doses of hydrochlorothiazide don't seem to lower the blood pressure any better than low doses.**

   Propranolol has proven itself in clinical trials, so start it at 20 mg twice daily.

Some physicians recommend starting with a drug combination (like propranolol hydrochloride and hydrochlorothiazide tablets) and not bothering with Step 1. But if the blood pressure is only mildly elevated, this initial combination isn't necessary.

Treating complicated high blood pressure

A number of complications may cause you to stop the diuretics and try a drug that can manage both the high blood pressure and the complication. The most important of these complications and their treatment are as follows:

- ✔ **Chest pain due to disease in the coronary arteries along with high blood pressure** responds better to beta blockers or calcium channel blockers.

- ✔ **Diabetes mellitus with kidney disease and high blood pressure** is best managed by an ACE inhibitor or one of the angiotensin II receptor blockers.

- ✔ **Fat abnormalities in the blood along with high blood pressure** are better treated with beta blockers that don't cause further fat abnormalities.

- ✔ **Hand tremors along with high blood pressure** may respond better to certain beta blockers like propranolol or nadolol.

- ✔ **Heart attacks with high blood pressure** respond better to a beta blocker and an ACE inhibitor as the first choice.

- ✔ **Heart failure** is best treated by an ACE inhibitor and a diuretic. This diuretic should be a more powerful loop diuretic (not a thiazide diuretic) because too much fluid in the body is one of the major problems.

- ✔ **Heart rhythm abnormalities with high blood pressure** do better on beta blockers or calcium channel blockers like verapamil or diltiazem, but not nifedipine.

- ✔ **Hyperthyroidism with high blood pressure** does best with a beta blocker.

- ✔ **Migraine headaches and high blood pressure** respond better to certain beta blockers (propranolol or nadolol) or calcium channel blockers (verapamil or diltiazem).

- ✔ **Surgery is safer** for the high blood pressure patient who uses a beta blocker during surgery.

Moving ahead when the first choice fails

If a prescription can't keep the blood pressure consistently under 140/90 mm Hg, further action must be taken:

- ✔ If the blood pressure doesn't respond or the side effects are intolerable, a drug from another class is given.

  If the diuretics and beta blockers can't be used, the next step is an ACE inhibitor.

- ✔ If the blood pressure is only partially controlled, a second drug from another drug class is added.

  If a diuretic hasn't been added, it should be added at this point.

- ✔ If the blood pressure still isn't under 140/90 mm Hg, a third drug is added.

You should see your doctor again within one month after a change in medication.

Even if you need several drugs to bring your blood pressure under control, this doesn't necessarily mean you'll be taking all these drugs the rest of your life. If you can lose weight or use some other method from Chapters 8 through 12 to bring down your blood pressure without drugs, you may be able to reduce dosages or stop some of the drugs. After a year of control (even without other improvements) and under your doctor's care, try to cut down on some of the drugs.

The goal blood pressure for a person with diabetes or kidney disease is even lower than 120/80 mm Hg.

Making sure you take your medicine

After becoming an expert on medications for high blood pressure and the right pill under the right circumstances, surely you plan to take each and every pill, right? What's that? You say that you have trouble remembering sometimes? Here are some suggestions to make your pill-taking second nature:

✔ Get into the habit of taking the pills at the same time each day.

✔ Associate your pill-taking with another task like brushing your teeth.

✔ Take pills that must be taken with food at the same meal each day.

✔ Get a plastic pillbox with a compartment for each day of the week; fill it at the beginning of each week.

✔ Put notes all over the house to remind you to take them.

✔ Set a pill pager to beep when you need to take your pills.

If you forget to take a dose, don't double the next dose! Just pick up where you left off as though you had taken the medication.

Recognizing Drug Side Effects

Being aware of side effects is important. The drugs in this chapter are great, but they're not perfect; they all cause side effects, and some of them are so severe that the patient must discontinue the drug. If you notice an uncomfortable change shortly after you start a new drug for high blood pressure, you can easily recognize which drug is to blame. But sometimes the side effect doesn't become apparent until months after you start the drug. At other times, the addition of another drug (for example, one that's treating another disease) brings out the side effect of the first drug.

The following list matches many of these side effects to the blood pressure drugs that are likely to cause them.

Side Effect	Drug That May Cause It
Anemia	Methyldopa
Breast enlargement	Spironolactone
Confusion	All diuretics
Constipation	Calcium channel blockers and diuretics

Decreased good cholesterol	Beta blockers
Decreased white blood cells	ACE inhibitors
Depression	Clonidine, guanabenz, guanfacine, and calcium channel blockers
Diarrhea	Potassium-sparing diuretics and beta blockers
Dizziness	All diuretics, labetalol, and doxazosin
Drowsiness	Alpha and beta blockers
Dry cough	ACE inhibitors
Dry eyes	Clonidine, guanabenz, and guanfacine
Dry mouth	All diuretics, methyldopa, clonidine, guanabenz, and guanfacine
Fatigue	Beta blockers and doxazosin
Fever	Methyldopa and labetalol
Fluid in breasts	Methyldopa and spironolactone
Headache	Vasodilators, calcium channel blockers, and ACE inhibitors
Heart failure	Alpha-1 adrenergic receptor antagonists and vasodilators
Increased asthma	Beta blockers and diuretics
Increased blood sugar	All diuretics and beta blockers
Increased cholesterol	Thiazide diuretics
Increased hairiness	Spironolactone and minoxidil
Increased urination	All diuretics and beta blockers
Insomnia and sleep disorders	Beta blockers
Irritation of the esophagus	Calcium channel blockers
Liver damage	Methyldopa
Loss of hearing	Loop diuretics
Loss of taste	ACE inhibitors
Lupus syndrome	Hydralazine
Menstrual irregularities	Spironolactone
Muscle pains	All diuretics
Nausea and vomiting	All diuretics

Rapid heart beat	Vasodilators
Reduced erections	Thiazide diuretics, spironolactone, and methyldopa
Sensitivity to cold	Alpha and beta blockers
Sensitivity to sunlight	Beta blockers and diuretics
Skin rashes	All diuretics and ACE inhibitors
Sleepiness	Methyldopa, clonidine, guanabenz, and guanfacine
Swelling of the abdomen	Potassium-sparing diuretics
Swelling of the legs	Vasodilators and calcium channel blockers
Swollen, tender gums	Calcium channel blockers
Thirst	All diuretics
Upset stomach	Beta blockers, diuretics, and angiotensin II receptor blockers
Very low blood pressure	ACE inhibitors
Vivid dreams or nightmares	Clonidine, guanabenz, guanfacine, and beta blockers
Weakness	All diuretics

If a side effect in this list describes how you're feeling, discuss it with your doctor and consider a reduction in dosage or a change in the medication to a different class of drugs.

Many other less-common problems are not listed here. If you have an unusual new symptom after starting a drug for high blood pressure, by all means, discuss it with your doctor and consider a reduction in dose or a change in medication.

In general, drugs in the same class have the same side effects. To rid yourself of an annoying side effect, you have to switch to a new class.

Identifying Brand Names

So many drugs, so many brand names. How can you know what you're on, much less what it does and what its side effects may be? Doctors more often refer to a drug by its brand name because remembering the brand name is easier than remembering the scientific name. The drug companies also want doctors to think of their drug when they write a prescription, so they give the drug a name that sticks in the mind, for example *lotensin*. Unfortunately, the brand name identifies the drug's effect but not its class.

In this section, I provide all the brand names of the current drugs in alphabetical order. To find a scientific name, just look up a brand name — its scientific name is in the right column. You may discover that you're on a drug that you shouldn't be on, or it may explain that irritating symptom you've been having.

Always keep an up-to-date list of *all* your drugs, preferably by scientific *and* brand name. Also list the frequency, the number of pills, and the milligrams of each pill you take. This record can save your doctor plenty of time when you need prescription renewals, and it helps any new doctor know more about your health.

Some of these drugs are no longer made under their brand name because the patent has run out; competing against the generic form of the drug is no longer profitable for the drug company. However, if your doctor is still using the brand name, you'll need to know it as well as its scientific name.

Brand Name	Scientific Name
Accupril	Quinapril
Accuretic	Quinapril and hydrochlorothiazide
Aceon	Perindopril
Adalat	Nifedipine
Aldactazide	Spironolactone and hydrochlorothiazide
Aldactone	Spironolactone
Aldoclor	Methyldopa and chlorothiazide
Aldomet	Methyldopa
Aldoril	Methyldopa and hydrochlorothiazide
Altace	Ramipril
Apresoline	Hydralazine
Apresozide	Hydralazine and hydrochlorothiazide
Atacand	Candesartan
Avalide	Irbesartan and hydrochlorothiazide
Avapro	Irbesartan
Benicar	Olmesartan and benicar HCT
Blocardren	Timolol
Bumex	Bumetanide

Calan	Verapamil
Capoten	Captopril
Capozide	Captopril and hydrochlorothiazide
Cardene SR	Nicardipine
Cardizem	Diltiazem
Cardizem CD	Diltiazem
Cardura	Doxazosin
Cardura XL	Doxazosin
Cartia XT	Diltiazem
Catapres	Clonidine
Clorpres	Clonidine and chlorthalidone
Corgard	Nadolol
Coreg	Carvedilol
Corzide	Nadolol and bendroflumethiazide
Covera	Verapamil
Cozaar	Losartan
Demadex	Torsemide
Dilacor XR	Diltiazem
Dilt CD	Diltiazem
Diltia XT	Diltiazem
Diovan	Valsartan
Diovan HCT	Valsartan and hydrochlorothiazide
Diuril Oral Suspension	Chlorothiazide
Diuril Tablets	Chlorothiazide
Dyazide	Triamterene and hydrochlorothiazide
Dyrenium	Triamterene
Edecrin	Ethacrynic acid
HydroDIURIL	Hydrochlorothiazide
Hygroton	Chlorthalidone
Hytrin	Terazosin
Hyzaar	Losartan and hydrochlorothiazide

Inderal	Propranolol
Inderide	Propranolol and hydrochlorothiazide
InnoPran XL	Propranolol
Isoptin	Verapamil
Lasix	Furosemide
Levatol	Penbutolol
Lexxel	Felodipine and enalapril
Loniten	Minoxidil
Lopressor	Metoprolol
Lotensin	Benazepril
Lotrel	Amlodipine and benazepril
Mavik	Trandolapril
Maxide	Triamterene and hydrochlorothiazide
Midamor	Amiloride
Minipress	Prazosin
Miscardis	Telmisartan
Miscardis XCT	Telmisartan and hydrochlorothiazide
Moduretic	Amiloride and hydrochlorothiazide
Monopril	Fosinopril
Mykrox	Metolazone
Naturetin	Bendroflumethiazide
Norvasc	Amlodipine
Oretic	Hydrochlorothiazide
Plendil	Felodipine
Prinivil	Lisinopril
Prinzide	Lisinopril and hydrochlorothiazide
Procardia	Nifedipine
Renese	Polythiazide
Sectral	Acebutolol
Sular	Nisoldipine
Tarka	Trandolapril and verapamil

Taztia XT	Diltiazem
Teczem	Diltiazem and enalapril
Tenex	Guanfacine
Tenormine	Atenolol
Teveten	Eprosartan
Thalitone	Chlorthalidone
Tiazac	Diltiazem
Timolide	Timolol and hydrochlorothiazide
Toprol XL	Metoprolol
Trandate	Labetalol
Uniretic	Moexipril and hydrochlorothiazide
Univasc	Moexipril
Vasotec	Enalapril
Verelan	Verapamil
Wytensin	Guanabenz
Zaroxolyn	Metolazone
Zebeta	Bisoprolol
Zestril	Lisinopril
Zestoretic	Lisinopril and hydrochlorothiazide
Ziac	Bisoprolol and hydrochlorothiazide

Part IV
Taking Care of Special Populations

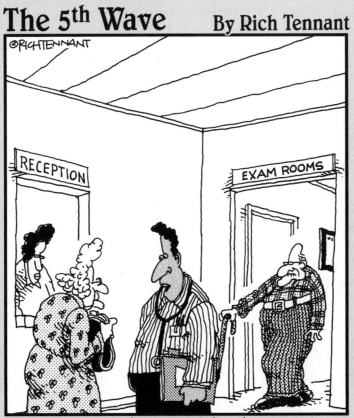

The 5th Wave   By Rich Tennant

RECEPTION   EXAM ROOMS

"Sometimes a tightness in the chest can be a sign of high blood pressure. In your husband's case, however, I just loosened his belt a little."

In this part . . .

Certain groups that may get high blood pressure require their own discussion. Certainly children, the elderly, and the pregnant female have so many of their own issues that they deserve separate treatment. If you or a loved one is in one of these groups, Part IV offers you everything you need to know about high blood pressure.

Chapter 14

Helping the Elderly

• •

• •

*W*ho are the *elderly?* It's a moving definition because more and more people are living longer and remaining healthier for a longer time. For the purposes of this chapter, I consider the start of *elder* years to be age 65. The elderly are growing in numbers. In the year 2000, one in eight Americans were elderly, but by 2030, one in five (about 70 million) Americans will fit that category. In addition to the growing population, the number of people living past 100 years of age is also climbing. So, over the next 30 years, the concerns of the elderly will become a major challenge throughout the world. Don't be surprised if bathing suit ads start featuring 70-year-old grandmothers instead of 17-year-old girls!

The elderly are different from the mainstream population (although I'm looking more and more like them). Of course, some elderly are quite healthy, but in general, they

✔ Usually have more than one disease

✔ May have a certain amount of memory loss, which makes taking pills more challenging

✔ Are often on multiple medications with all the problems of drug interactions

✔ May not have as good nutrition as they did at an earlier age

✔ May have lost some kidney function

✔ May have poor vision

The elderly are also at the greatest risk of a brain attack (see Chapter 7) or a heart attack (see Chapter 5), but controlling their blood pressure reduces this risk by up to 25 percent. A study in the February 1992 *British Medical Journal* showed that using medication for high blood pressure in the elderly between the ages of 65 and 74 reduced the occurrence of brain attacks by 25 percent and heart attacks by 17 percent.

The incidence of high blood pressure among the elderly is enormous. Among individuals 75 years and older, 75 percent of women and 65 percent of men have high blood pressure.

As I write this, the Hypertension in the Very Elderly Trial (a key study in England) is in progress, researching the effect that blood pressure control has on the health of people 80 years and older. The pilot study of 1,283 patients, published in the December 2003 *Journal of Hypertension,* showed a definite reduction in brain attacks and heart attacks. However, it also raised a question of excessive overall deaths in the actively treated patients compared to the patients given placebos. (The placebos should have had no effect on blood pressure.) The final report will be out soon.

But plenty of information is available now to support the claim that blood pressure control does indeed affect the health of the elderly for the better. Whether you're elderly or you have a loved one who is elderly with high blood pressure, I suggest you don't wait for the results of that study to bring that blood pressure under control. And read this chapter; it can help you understand and approach the special problems of high blood pressure in the elderly.

Evaluating Mental Ability

If a question exists about an elderly person's ability to take medications, feed himself properly, and get physical exercise, then evaluating his mental ability is important. This step can be a brief mental-status examination by a doctor to evaluate the following abilities:

- Orientation in time (day and year) and space (city and state)
- Ability to repeat items, read, write, draw, calculate, name items, and remember items previously named
- Comprehension

Standard versions of this test give an individual score; a perfect score is 30. One version is the Mini-Mental State Examination, which takes only ten minutes. A person who scores less than 26 probably has some mental disability that can be further tested. This is a good baseline test for any elderly person, not just for one with high blood pressure, and it can be repeated at intervals to observe deterioration. The test can also help determine whether a loss of mental acuity is due to medication.

Your doctor should perform a brief mental-status examination on your loved one at every office visit to look for indications that she can't care for herself. The Abbreviated Mental Test Score takes a minute or two, and it's an excellent routine test for ongoing testing of mental acuity. You can do it at home as well.

If some degree of mental acuity is lost, then you shouldn't expect the elderly individual to be responsible for her own medical care (especially the administration of drugs). You or a healthcare professional — at home, in an assisted living facility, or in a nursing home — must take charge of medical care.

Assessing Blood Pressure

In the highly industrialized countries of the world, the populations' systolic blood pressure rises throughout life. In contrast, the diastolic blood pressure begins to level off around age 55 or 60 and often falls after this leveling off occurs. This diastolic drop is the result of increasing stiffness of arteries with aging. (See Chapter 2 for the basics on systolic and diastolic blood pressure.)

Changes in an elderly person's blood pressure may have an unknown cause or result from a disease. Other factors such as medications may also cause his blood pressure to rise. I tell you what you need to know about these scenarios in the following sections.

Dealing with essential high blood pressure

Almost all high blood pressure in the elderly is *essential* (high blood pressure for which the cause is unknown). Most of the high blood pressure in the elderly is also *isolated systolic high blood pressure* (the systolic blood pressure is over 140 mm Hg, but the diastolic blood pressure is less than 90 mm Hg). In the elderly, systolic blood pressure can predict a brain attack or a heart attack. In contrast, their diastolic blood pressure elevation doesn't suggest the same risks as it does in a younger person. Most often, *isolated diastolic high blood pressure* (the systolic blood pressure is less than 140 mm Hg, but the diastolic blood pressure is greater than 90 mm Hg) poses no risk among the elderly. ***Note:*** An individual whose isolated diastolic blood pressure is greater than 105 mm Hg probably needs some treatment, especially when complications of high blood pressure are present.

The tricky business of detecting pseudo high blood pressure

Pseudo high blood pressure is a condition resulting from the calcification of the arteries. Due to aging, calcium begins to deposit along the artery and can lead to an inaccurate blood pressure reading (the artery doesn't compress when the cuff around the arm is inflated). Even though the blood pressure inside the artery is normal, the blood pressure meter registers high (as much as 20 to 30 mm Hg higher than its true value). A few clues can indicate this condition:

✔ No other signs of a high blood pressure complication

✔ Little change in blood pressure despite adequate treatment

✔ Low blood pressure symptoms despite normal or even high measured blood pressure

A doctor can use other techniques to get a direct measurement of blood pressure and thereby evaluate the possibility of pseudo high blood pressure.

If you or a loved one is over 65 years of age with a systolic blood pressure reading that's greater than 140 on several occasions, you need some treatment, lifestyle changes, or medication to bring it down. Get together with your physician to set up a treatment plan.

Most of the time, an elderly person discovers that she has high blood pressure during a routine examination or as part of a screening program by a local hospital or drugstore. However, about 10 percent of long-standing high blood pressure cases are first diagnosed when a serious complication like a brain attack or a heart attack occurs.

For some reason, elderly women don't seem to receive adequate treatment as often as elderly men. Make sure your mother is checked and treated!

Considering secondary high blood pressure

Secondary high blood pressure means the high blood pressure is a direct result of a specific disease or disorder. If the disease disappears or is treated, then the high blood pressure usually lowers. (Chapter 4 covers the various causes of secondary high blood pressure.) Even though an elderly person's high blood pressure is rarely (probably less than 1 percent) due to another disease, you should consider the possibility of secondary high blood pressure (and therefore its possible cure) under the following circumstances:

- ✔ Newly developed high blood pressure beyond 60 years of age
- ✔ Failure of three or more blood pressure drugs to control the blood pressure
- ✔ Symptoms or lab findings that suggest secondary high blood pressure
- ✔ A low potassium level before taking drugs or when the patient takes a small dose of a *thiazide diuretic* (see Chapter 13 for more about this type of drug)
- ✔ Continuing evidence of kidney function loss despite adequate blood pressure control

The steps to evaluate and treat the patient are in Chapter 4. ***Note:*** Unless it developed recently, secondary high blood pressure in the elderly usually doesn't lower even when the cause is eliminated because

- ✔ The high blood pressure has often been present for a long time.
- ✔ The elderly also tend to have essential high blood pressure.

Examining the meds that elevate blood pressure in the elderly

Many elderly suffer from arthritis and receive *nonsteroidal anti-inflammatory drugs* (NSAIDs). New NSAIDs come along on an almost daily basis, but the most common pain-reducing medications (with their brand names in parentheses) as of this writing include

- ✔ Aspirin in high doses (two aspirin three or more times a day)
- ✔ Celecoxib (Celebrex)
- ✔ Diclofenac (Voltaren)
- ✔ Diflunisal (Dolobid)
- ✔ Etodolac (Lodine)
- ✔ Ibuprofen (Motrin, Advil)
- ✔ Indomethacin (Indocin)

- ✔ Nabumetone (Relafen)
- ✔ Naproxen (Naprosyn)
- ✔ Oxaprozin (Daypro)
- ✔ Piroxicam (Feldene)
- ✔ Sulindac (Clinoril); see the *Tip* following this list

An elderly person with high blood pressure taking an NSAID should discontinue the NSAID if possible, but only after consulting with his physician. These drugs, especially when mixed with drugs for high blood pressure, block the action of the high blood pressure drug and raise the blood pressure.

Of the NSAIDs, sulindac has been shown *not* to cause an increase in high blood pressure or to oppose the effect of blood pressure medications. This may be the drug of choice when an elderly individual — particularly one with high blood pressure — needs an NSAID.

Another factor is the *white coat effect* (see Chapter 2), which is much greater in the elderly than the younger population. The white coat effect means that your systolic blood pressure may be 10 mm Hg higher when a physician takes the reading as compared to when you take your blood pressure at home. An elderly patient may even have high blood pressure in the doctor's office and low blood pressure at home. For this reason, home blood pressure monitoring is a good idea for the elderly; it helps determine whether their treatment is excessive or sufficient. I explain how to monitor blood pressure at home in Chapter 2.

As the kidneys go, so goes the blood pressure

In a normal, healthy person, blood flow to the kidney decreases about 10 percent each decade after age 30. So more than likely, the diminishing function of one or both kidneys is responsible for high blood pressure in the elderly. And this circulation to the kidney declines further when high blood pressure, diabetes, or heart failure is present.

The main consequence of decreased blood flow to the kidney is the kidney's decreased ability to get rid of the body's salt and water. This salt and water buildup causes the blood pressure to rise, which further decreases the kidney function. It's a vicious cycle.

The elderly also experience problems in the walls of their blood vessels. Over time, the production of nitric oxide (the most important chemical relaxant for the muscular walls of the arteries) is reduced; its absence leads to higher blood pressure.

Epinephrine and norepinephrine (hormones from the adrenal gland, see Chapter 4) tend to be elevated in an elderly person's blood and don't fall (as they normally should) as blood pressure rises. They contribute to high blood pressure by raising blood pressure, heart rate, and blood glucose.

Improving Nutrition to Lower Blood Pressure

The goal of nutrition among the elderly is to provide the right amount of kilocalories with enough vitamins and minerals from the appropriate energy sources. By cutting calories and eating foods full of nutrients, the elderly can vastly improve their blood pressure.

Shopping with an elderly person in a supermarket may help you emphasize the valuable information on food labels regarding the salt content in food products. Point out the best choices, which are usually also the freshest foods.

In the following sections, I explain how to evaluate an elderly person's diet and give tips on changing a diet for the better.

Assessing diet

A dietary assessment determines whether an elderly person is getting enough of the right foods. One simple technique is to ask the person to write down everything he eats for three days. A complementary method is to ask him to record how many times he eats a particular kind of food in a day, a week, or a month. However, his memory may limit the accuracy of these approaches. In this case, a doctor can also measure blood levels of minerals and vitamins to determine whether these nutrients are present in adequate amounts.

A dietary assessment may turn up the following concerns in an elderly individual's diet:

- Low vitamin and mineral intake
- Low fresh vegetable and fresh fruit intake
- Little variety in the diet
- Excessive salt intake
- Insufficient calories
- Frequent complaints of illness

The elderly with insufficient diets are often poor and uneducated, but inadequate diets are also found among the well to do.

Because of the high cost of drugs, many elderly claim that they must choose between good nutrition and their drugs. Although this economic problem is beyond the scope of this book, it's an important consideration. To be effective, high blood pressure treatment for the elderly must address both nutrition and drugs.

Following the DASH diet

Elderly people who follow the DASH diet that I describe in Chapter 9 may reduce their blood pressure enough to eliminate a blood pressure medication. And because the side effects of drugs and drug interactions are a special problem in this population, eliminating a drug is a goal worth achieving.

Additional benefits of the DASH diet include the following:

- ✔ It's low in saturated fat and cholesterol. Reducing these two dangers also contributes to the reduction of brain attacks and heart attacks in the elderly.
- ✔ It reduces kilocalorie intake. Because energy needs decline with age, the DASH diet is a great way to curb those calories while lowering blood pressure enormously and reducing the risk of a heart attack.

Reducing salt intake

Eating fresh foods and using herbs and spices in place of salt are essential for the elderly, who are more sensitive to the blood-pressure-raising effect of salt than younger people. The lower the salt intake, the lower the blood pressure.

When the DASH diet accompanies a reduction in salt intake, the result is even greater. In fact, many elderly who follow DASH and reduce salt can avoid all blood pressure medications. But reducing salt can be especially difficult for several reasons:

- ✔ Because age reduces taste sensation, the elderly may compensate by adding more salt to food.
- ✔ The elderly may live alone and not be able to consume fresh food before it spoils. As a result, they need to rely on prepared foods that contain salt. In addition, the elderly also tend to consume more prepared foods, which can be a major source of salt intake.
- ✔ They may lack the energy or ability to put a healthy meal together.

Head to Chapter 10 for plenty of tips on keeping salt out of your diet.

Changing the Lifestyle to Lower Blood Pressure

Just as reducing salt intake tends to lower an elderly person's blood pressure more than a younger individual's, lifestyle changes also tend to lower an elderly person's blood pressure more than a younger person's. The most important changes include the following:

- ✔ Reducing alcohol intake is essential (see Chapter 11).

- ✔ Quitting tobacco is beneficial at any age (see Chapter 11).

- ✔ Reducing excessive caffeine intake (more than two cups of regular coffee daily; see Chapter 11) is helpful.

- ✔ Increasing daily exercise lowers blood pressure but also benefits the older person in many other ways (for example, reducing the chance of a fall, helping with weight loss, and adding strength to perform the tasks of daily living; see Chapter 12).

- ✔ Incorporating a yoga program, meditation, or biofeedback may reduce blood pressure (see Chapter 12).

Adding lifestyle changes to the proper diet goes a long way toward eliminating the need for drugs. The March 1998 *Journal of the American Medical Association* presented a study (the Trial of Nonpharmacologic Interventions in the Elderly) in which 975 men and women with high blood pressure between the ages of 60 and 80 were divided into four groups:

- ✔ **Salt reduction:** 1,800 mg of salt daily

- ✔ **Weight loss:** At least a ten-pound weight loss

- ✔ **Salt reduction and weight loss:** A combination of the salt-reduction and weight-loss groups

- ✔ **Control:** No special restrictions

After three months, 30 percent of the entire group stopped all blood pressure medications. The results showed:

- ✔ The combined group (salt reduction and weight loss) did best in lowering blood pressure.

- ✔ Both the salt-reduction group and the weight-loss group did much better than the control group.

A key result is that the lifestyle changes lasted up to three years after the end of the study in these patients, even after decades of physical inactivity and unhealthy eating habits.

The National Long-term Care Survey (check it out on the Internet at www. nltcs.aas.duke.edu/index.htm) paints an optimistic picture of disability, including high blood pressure, among the elderly in the future. The survey has studied 35,000 to 40,000 Americans at intervals of two to five years since 1982. The unexpected finding is that *chronic disability* (the inability to do daily living activities like brushing teeth, shaving, dressing, and cleaning) among the elderly is falling. The statistics show

- Between 1982 and 1989, the prevalence of chronic disability fell at the rate of 1 percent per year.
- Between 1989 and 1994, it fell at 1.6 percent per year.
- Between 1994 and 1999, it fell at 2.6 percent per year.
- Between 1999 and 2004, it fell at 1.4 percent per year.

If the prevalence of chronic disability continues to lower, the 2040 statistic will be 50 percent of the 2000 one. And this improvement means that despite a huge gain in the elderly population, the total number of disabled will be the same in 2040 as the year 2000. The main reasons for this falling rate of chronic disability are

- The adoption of lifestyle changes among the elderly population
- The use of medical intervention

This reminds me of an unlikely couple: an 80-year-old man who fell in love with a 20-year-old woman. She insisted that they get their health checked before considering marriage, and a doctor, after examining them both, told them they were in excellent health. "However," said the doctor, "I'm concerned about the age difference." The future husband replied, "Well, what can you do? If she dies, she dies."

Taking Drugs to Lower Blood Pressure

Some patients are unwilling or unable to make lifestyle changes. Even if they do change their habits, some patients still need to take drugs to lower their blood pressure to a safer level that doesn't cause illness or death. A number of basic recommendations are especially pertinent to these folks:

- ✔ An elderly person should take medication when the systolic blood pressure is 160 mm Hg or greater.

  The zone between 140 and 160 mm Hg is a gray area. Elderly people without complications of high blood pressure whose blood pressure is less than 160 mm Hg may not benefit from treatment. However, when damage to the heart or blood vessels or a history of a brain attack is evident, then blood pressures between 140 and 160 mm Hg should also be treated with drugs.

- ✔ Drug treatment should continue regardless of age so long as the patient is expected to live and side effects are mild.

- ✔ In the elderly, diuretics like *hydrochlorothiazide* are the drug of first choice despite the presence of other conditions such as heart disease or diabetes.

- ✔ A once-daily medication is preferable to divided doses in order to keep the regimen simple and therefore successful.

- ✔ An elderly person should start with half the usual beginning dose and then make changes slowly as he becomes acclimated to the drug.

- ✔ Make sure the elderly individual can open the medication bottle and understands how to take the medication. Some safety bottles are impossible to open for people who have arthritis or vision problems.

- ✔ Drug interactions are a major potential problem because the elderly may be taking a number of prescription drugs. An elderly person should work with his physician at every visit to try to reduce the number of drugs he takes.

In the following sections, I walk you through medication choices for elderly people with high blood pressure. See Chapter 13 for the full scoop on drug therapy.

Primary drug therapy: Thiazide diuretic

If an elderly person has uncomplicated high blood pressure, the first medication choice is a thiazide diuretic. *Note:* This is the same drug that a younger person without complications takes, but the elderly person should take half the usual dose. A dose of 12.5 mg of hydrochlorothiazide is effective in most elderly people. Going up to 50 mg is rarely necessary.

Although high doses of a thiazide diuretic can raise cholesterol (the elderly often have high cholesterol, a harmful blood fat), a low dose probably has little effect on the cholesterol.

If an elderly person's potassium or sodium level is already low or her calcium is high, she can take a drug that combines a thiazide diuretic with a potassium-sparing drug. *Note:* Potassium supplements aren't recommended for the elderly because the individual may have trouble taking them by mouth and eliminating the excess by the kidney.

Second choice: Beta blocker

If the patient can't take a thiazide diuretic, *a beta blocker* is the second choice. Beta blockers aren't as effective as thiazide diuretics and are associated with more side effects.

Beta blockers are less useful in elderly people who have asthma, chronic lung disease, or severe obstructive disease of the blood vessels. When the thiazide diuretic doesn't completely control the blood pressure, the addition of a beta blocker often accomplishes a satisfactory level.

Third-choice drugs

Calcium channel blockers, ACE inhibitors, and *angiotensin II receptor blockers* aren't as effective as a thiazide diuretic or a beta blocker, but the elderly can take them when thiazide diuretics and beta blockers aren't appropriate for some reason (like an allergy to the drugs). These third-choice drugs definitely lower the blood pressure, but they haven't been shown to reduce illness and death due to high blood pressure.

Medications for the treatment of high blood pressure can pose several dangers including the following:

- The initial dose of an ACE inhibitor must be reduced for an elderly person. If the usual starting dose is 10 mg, it should be 5 mg for the elderly person.

- When an ACE inhibitor is added to a diuretic, *low* blood pressure becomes a great danger — especially in the elderly. As a precaution, the diuretic should be stopped for a few days before the ACE inhibitor is added.

- The other classes of drugs that act on the brain (like *methyldopa, clonidine, guanfacine,* and *guanabenz* as well as the *alpha adrenergic receptor blockers*) have limited use among the elderly population. These powerful agents cause drowsiness and depression; the drop in blood pressure when standing can be dangerous.

Special situations

Because chest pain associated with heart disease is so common in the elderly, a beta blocker is an appropriate first choice of treatment for high blood pressure when the elderly person also has chest pain due to coronary atherosclerosis (see Chapter 5).

ACE inhibitors have been shown to prolong the lives of people with congestive heart failure; they are the drugs of choice when heart failure accompanies high blood pressure.

ACE inhibitors and angiotensin II receptor blockers are especially good for the elderly person with high blood pressure and kidney disease (often associated with diabetes).

Avoiding Dangerous Falls in Blood Pressure

Ten percent of the elderly population may experience *postural hypotension* (a sudden, dramatic fall in blood pressure of 20 mm Hg or more after standing as compared to sitting down). When the elderly have systolic high blood pressure, diabetes, or adrenal gland failure, the frequency of these large falls in blood pressure on standing is even greater. The symptoms may include blurred vision, lightheadedness, dizziness, and even a loss of consciousness.

Two tendencies account for postural hypotension in the elderly:

✔ Blood tends to remain in the lower part of the body because of a loss of muscle tone and a loss of valves in blood vessels that ordinarily prevent blood backflow.

✔ Elderly people sometimes lose the normal response of certain pressure sensors in the neck that detect falling blood pressure. When functioning properly, these sensors signal the heart to pump more blood into the brain. The heart pumps harder and other blood vessels constrict to push blood back to the heart. However, when the sensors aren't functioning, the decreased blood in the brain may lead to a fainting spell or dizziness. *Note:* The increase of blood in the intestinal blood vessels after eating may contribute to the reduction in blood flow to the brain.

A number of approaches treat falls in blood pressure on standing. Some of them include

- ✔ Tilting the bed to elevate the person's head
- ✔ Wearing elastic hose that reduce pooling of blood in the legs
- ✔ Performing leg exercises to push blood back to the heart
- ✔ Testing for and treating possible dehydration
- ✔ Adding adrenal medication to restore hormones after adrenal failure
- ✔ Reducing the dose of blood pressure medication, particularly beta blockers and alpha blockers
- ✔ Sometimes controlling the blood pressure with drugs may reduce the tendency for a fall in blood pressure. Certain drugs stimulate the blood vessels to contract, thus raising the blood pressure.

Chapter 15

Handling High Blood Pressure in Children

Children, like the elderly, are different from you and me. They're much smaller and still growing. Children are tuned in to the opinions of their peers and usually don't like to be different. Having a chronic disease like high blood pressure makes them stand out, and they don't want to. As a result, they may be unwilling to take the necessary steps to manage their blood pressure — dieting and losing weight, reducing salt, and taking medications.

Adult high blood pressure is much more common in people who had the problem as children. And just as high blood pressure is more common in black adults, it is also much more common in black children. Nevertheless, high blood pressure used to be a rare event in children. Before 1980, less than 2 percent of children in the United States under the age of 18 had high blood pressure. Now, more than 5 percent of that population have been diagnosed with it. And although childhood high blood pressure may have a number of causes, the major reason for its increase is the increase in childhood weight problems and obesity.

A child is considered *overweight* if he's heavier than 85 percent of the children of the same age and height. The child is *obese* if he's heavier than 95 percent of the children of the same age and height. Check out the charts your child's doctor has that relate weight to age and height, or go to the following Web site to find growth charts: www.keepkidshealthy.com/growthcharts.

If your child's blood pressure is checked periodically, you can find out plenty even though there isn't a persistent increase in high blood pressure. Many experts believe that the roots of adult high blood pressure are established in childhood. So if these early signs can be detected and managed early enough, adult high blood pressure may be prevented.

In this chapter, you find all the information you need to help prevent high blood pressure in your child or manage it if your child already has it. (For the purposes of this chapter, children range in age from newborn to age 18.) Reward, praise, and encourage your child's positive efforts, however small, rather than punish your child for *not* doing what she should.

Consider the example of the minister who needed his congregation to contribute more money to rebuild the church. He said to his parishioners, "Anyone willing to donate for the church fund, please stand up." At that precise moment, the organist broke out with a rousing rendition of the "Star Spangled Banner." The congregation felt good about standing for the national anthem *and* the minister got his volunteers!

Measuring Blood Pressure Correctly

Just as in adults, proper measurement of a child's blood pressure is essential to make a correct diagnosis. But this step can be especially challenging when the small child is *unenthusiastic* about having his arm wrapped in a cuff and squeezed while a stranger holds an instrument against his arm. The following sections show you how to accomplish a proper blood pressure reading in any child; head to Chapter 2 for the basics of measuring blood pressure.

Using Doppler ultrasound on tiny arms

Diagnosing high blood pressure is different for children. Measuring blood pressure with a stethoscope in the smallest infants and children is difficult because the sounds are so hard to hear in their tiny arms. To overcome this problem, pediatricians use *Doppler ultrasound* instruments to take blood pressure in the smallest arteries (usually in children under 3 years of age).

Doppler was an Austrian who discovered that sound has a different pitch when it comes toward you than when it goes away. If a sound wave is directed to an artery while a blood pressure cuff is cutting off the blood flow, the wave has one appearance. But when blood begins to flow through the artery as the cuff is deflated, the sound wave has a different appearance (this is the systolic blood pressure). As the cuff is opened further, the flow reaches its peak and the sound wave changes again (the diastolic blood pressure). The Doppler ultrasound instrument looks like a pencil that the doctor holds over the artery; it's connected to a machine that amplifies the sound waves so you can hear the distinct differences as the waves are altered by the blood flow.

Selecting the proper cuff size

The width of the blood pressure cuff must be appropriate for the size of the child's arm. If the cuff is too small, the reading will be too high. If the cuff is too large, the reading will be too low. The cuff has to completely surround the upper arm, but the length of the bladder — the part of the cuff that inflates with air — must also cover at least 80 percent of the circumference of the upper arm. Its width should also be 40 percent of the distance from the elbow to the shoulder.

If your child is between cuff sizes, use the larger cuff. A small cuff usually produces a falsely elevated reading, but a larger cuff usually doesn't change the reading enough to miss a high blood pressure reading.

Using proper technique

The doctor alters his technique for measuring the blood pressure depending on the age of your child. These guidelines help ensure an accurate reading:

- ✔ The child should have a chance to acclimate to the exam room before a blood pressure reading is taken.
- ✔ A baby should be lying quietly, not sucking or crying.
- ✔ In older children (usually age 3 and older), the doctor can use the stethoscope to measure the blood pressure in the conventional manner.
- ✔ Children old enough to sit usually prefer to sit rather than lie down.
- ✔ Whether the child is lying or sitting, the arm should be level with the heart.
- ✔ The right arm is conventionally used to measure children.
- ✔ If the blood pressure is elevated, the doctor should measure the blood pressure in both arms and the legs on that same visit.

Interpreting the Results of the Measurement

Children begin their lives with much lower blood pressure than they have later on. When you understand the normal progression of blood pressure in children, you can better recognize when their blood pressure is too high. In addition, height and weight must be taken into account because blood pressure is dependent on them.

The blood pressure of a newborn averages 70/45 mm Hg. Within a month, the systolic pressure rises to 85 mm Hg, and the blood pressure continues to rise throughout childhood. Table 15-1 shows the 95th percentile *(high-normal)* blood pressures — that is, the *maximum* normal blood pressures for different ages.

The 90th percentile blood pressures are generally 4 mm Hg lower than the 95th percentile numbers, both systolic and diastolic. For example, if 126/78 mm Hg is the 95th percentile for children ages 13 to 15, then 122/74 mm Hg is the 90th percentile. **Note:** Children with blood pressures between the 90th and the 95th percentile levels are *high normal.*

Table 15-1	Maximum Normal Blood Pressure at Different Ages
Age	*Blood Pressure*
Newborn	70/45 mm Hg
1 to 5 years	115/75 mm Hg
6 to 12 years	125/80 mm Hg
13 to 15 years	126/78 mm Hg
16 to 18 years	132/82 mm Hg
Over 18 years	139/89 mm Hg

Height can affect blood pressure. Normally, a taller child has higher blood pressure than a shorter child of the same age. The tallest child at age 10 may have a maximum blood pressure reading of 123/82 mm Hg while the shortest child at age 10 may have a maximum blood pressure reading of 114/77 mm Hg.

The 1987 Task Force Report from the National Institute of Health and the National Heart, Lung, and Blood Institute established tables for the *90th and 95th percentile blood pressure levels* for boys and girls ages 1 through 17 at various heights. Check out the tables at www.nhlbi.nih.gov/health/prof/heart/hbp/hbp_ped.htm and remember these distinctions:

- The *90th percentile* of blood pressure is the highest reading that 90 percent of children of the same sex, height, and age should have.

- Children with blood pressures less than the 90th percentile have *normal* blood pressures.

- Children with blood pressures between the 90th and 95th percentiles have *high-normal* blood pressures.

- Children over the *95th percentile* have *high* blood pressure and need to take steps to bring it down.

If your child has a blood pressure above the 90th percentile but 95th percentile, the blood pressure should be rechecked within thi months. Generally, the repeat blood pressures will be normal.

Children tend to be emotional in a doctor's office. The *white coat effect* is often the reason for a child's elevated blood pressure. Home monitoring of blood pressure may help to rule out this problem. See Chapter 2 for details.

Considering the Causes of Elevated Blood Pressure

Although the causes of high blood pressure in children vary, inheritance plays a role and so does disease. Some factors such as family history of high blood pressure can help identify children at high risk for high blood pressure as adults. The earlier that preventive measures are taken, the more likely the child will *not* develop high blood pressure, regardless of the cause. The future of quality high blood pressure care lies in prevention.

Surveying hereditary influences

Genetics undoubtedly influences the development of high blood pressure. If a parent has high blood pressure, one-third of her children are likely to develop it as well. If both parents have high blood pressure, two out of three children are likely to develop it.

Children who are likely to have high blood pressure as adults because their parents have high blood pressure may react differently to many challenges than children whose parents don't have high blood pressure. For example, children born to parents with high blood pressure may

- ✔ Have a greater rise in pulse rate than usual during exercise
- ✔ Experience an excessive rise in blood pressure after exercise
- ✔ Respond to emotional stress with a much greater rise in blood pressure
- ✔ Respond to a mental challenge like a school test with a rise in blood pressure
- ✔ Often have increased plasma renin activity (increased presence of a chemical that tends to raise blood pressure)

These abnormalities are especially striking in children from ethnic groups that have the highest prevalence of high blood pressure, especially African Americans (see Chapter 3 for more on groups at risk for high blood pressure).

Usually an adopted child doesn't develop high blood pressure even if both adoptive parents have it *unless* at least one biological parent also has it. If one identical twin has high blood pressure, the other has more than a 50-percent chance of also developing it. But if a fraternal twin has high blood pressure, the other has less than a 50-percent chance of developing it.

Factoring in weight

A strong relationship between weight and blood pressure exists at any age. But being overweight or obese during childhood is a significant factor of high blood pressure early in life and in the child's future. Consider these additional facts:

- A child who is breast-fed will generally have a lower-rate weight gain during infancy and lower blood pressure later in life than a child who is fed enriched formula.
- Newborns who have a low birth weight tend to have higher blood pressures by the time they're adolescents than those who have normal weight at birth.
- If an overweight child loses weight, she often reverses her high blood pressure.
- Even when the overweight condition doesn't continue into adulthood, the adult who was overweight as a child has a higher rate of heart illness as an adult.

  These children tend to eat more salt than their peers who are without high blood pressure.

Resulting from disease

When a newborn or a child up through 6 years of age has high blood pressure, it's usually *secondary* high blood pressure (the result of a disease). The most common causes in this age group are kidney disease, blockage of one or both arteries to the kidney, or *coarctation* (narrowing) of the aorta. I discuss these causes in Chapter 4.

Beginning at age 7, *essential* high blood pressure (high blood pressure for which the cause is unknown) begins to appear, although it's still rare at this age. Kidney disease and blockage of the kidney arteries are still frequent causes of secondary high blood pressure in this age group. Elevated blood pressure due to overweight and obese conditions also becomes important at this age.

Before age 11, up to 90 percent of the children with high blood pressure have secondary high blood pressure. By age 11, essential high blood pressure becomes more prevalent, and the causes begin to look more like adult causes.

Pinpointing the Cause of Your Child's Elevated Blood Pressure

If you discover that your child has high blood pressure, your child must undergo a careful evaluation. The cause is most often secondary to a known disease, which may be reversible. The doctor's evaluation should include a careful history of the child and the family, a physical examination emphasizing possible causes of high blood pressure, and appropriate laboratory studies that may point to a cause.

Noting key points in the child's history

Because of high blood pressure's hereditary connection, finding out whether high blood pressure is present in parents, grandparents, and close relatives is important. If brothers and sisters of the child also have high blood pressure, then a genetic basis for the high blood pressure may be established. A family history of obesity is also predictive of high blood pressure in the child.

The child may have a history of an illness that can damage the kidneys (repeated infections of the kidney or bladder, for example). An important clue to the cause of high blood pressure in the older child is the abuse of legal drugs like amphetamines or illegal drugs like cocaine. These drugs can be detected in blood tests.

Knowing what your child eats is essential. He may eat many packaged foods high in kilocalories and salt.

Uncovering clues during the physical examination

Getting an accurate pulse is also important because a rapid pulse rate may suggest an excess of certain hormones. An accurate height and weight allows the doctor to place the blood pressure in the correct percentile.

Of course, it's sometimes difficult to get the correct weight of a small child, but consider the clerk's suggestion in the story that follows:

At a pharmacy, a young woman asked to use the infant scale to weigh the baby in her arms. The clerk explained that the device was out for repairs, but he suggested that the mother could figure the infant's weight by first weighing herself with the baby on the adult scale and then weighing herself alone. To find the baby's weight, she just had to subtract the second weight from the first. "But that's impossible," countered the woman, "I'm not the mother; I'm the baby's aunt."

Other important features in the physical examination of the child from age 1 to 18 include the following:

- ✔ The blood pressure is taken in both arms and both legs (I discuss how to measure a child's blood pressure earlier in this chapter). A large difference suggests coarctation of the aorta.

- ✔ The physical appearance of the child may suggest a diagnosis of Cushing's syndrome (see Chapter 4). A round, flushed face and pigmented stretch marks may be present, for example.

- ✔ The doctor listens carefully for humming sounds over the arteries to the kidneys and the aorta. These sounds suggest obstruction to the flow of blood.

- ✔ A careful eye examination can show any changes associated with high blood pressure.

- ✔ The doctor carefully observes the size and feels the texture of the thyroid gland; abnormal function of this gland may be a cause of high blood pressure.

- ✔ The doctor examines the heart for damage due to high blood pressure, particularly enlargement; he is able to feel where the left side of the heart beats against the chest.

- ✔ He feels the abdomen for the presence of masses that suggest a tumor.

Getting help from the laboratory

If the doctor clearly suspects a secondary cause of high blood pressure, he can order the specific lab tests I note in Chapter 4. If no clear cause is found, the doctor can order several tests to narrow the diagnosis:

- ✔ Examination of the urine can reveal the infection that leads to kidney damage. A urine exam can also show the presence of blood and excess protein, which may indicate that the kidneys are leaking abnormally.

- ✔ An ultrasound study of the kidneys can show the size and shape of the kidneys as well as any appearance of disease. (Kidney damage is frequently the cause of secondary high blood pressure in younger children.)

- ✔ Blood levels of chemicals that are necessary for kidney function are helpful.

- ✔ A blood potassium level can help rule out a rare aldosterone-making tumor.

With a complete evaluation, a doctor can find the cause in most children. If the cause is reversible (such as obstruction of a kidney artery or coarctation of the aorta), then surgery is needed. The effects of irreversible causes (like a damaged kidney) can be slowed down by treating the high blood pressure with lifestyle changes and, when necessary, medication.

Beginning Treatment with Lifestyle Changes

Lifestyle changes can control high blood pressure. They may be all that's necessary to reverse high blood pressure in many children, especially older children. The various steps include the following:

- ✔ **Avoiding stress:** If stress is playing a role in the high blood pressure, this must be addressed. The child may need some brief therapy to deal with his fears and concerns about having a disease that none of his buddies have to deal with.

- ✔ **Choosing healthy foods:** Encourage the child to follow a diet that is low in fats but has more servings of fruits, vegetables, and grains. The DASH diet (see Chapter 9) lowers the blood pressure in the normal-weight child as well as the overweight child.

- ✔ **Controlling diabetes:** If the child has diabetes, controlling the blood glucose can help control blood pressure.

- ✔ **Exercising:** Exercise (see Chapter 12) is another key to lifelong high blood pressure prevention. The child needs to understand that moving the body is as crucial to lifelong health as eating properly. Some question exists about the relationship between strenuous exercise and high blood pressure in children. (Find out more about exercise in the following section.)

- ✔ **Losing weight:** If the child is overweight, great effort should be made to help the child lose weight by carefully evaluating the current diet and altering it. Suggestions include

    - Eliminating obvious sources of empty kilocalories like sodas

    - Reducing sources of saturated fat and cholesterol

    - Reducing portions of all foods to get the total kilocalorie intake low enough to produce a slow but steady weight loss

    Don't completely deprive the child of the joys of eating. In moderation, a hamburger or pizza can fit into a diet.

✔ **Quitting alcohol:** We know that alcohol raises blood pressure and stopping it causes a fall in blood pressure.

✔ **Quitting coffee:** A child who drinks coffee with caffeine should be encouraged to give it up. This habit easily continues in adulthood, so it's best to eliminate it at a young age. Don't forget about caffeine-containing soft drinks either. Chapter 11 has more information.

✔ **Quitting tobacco:** Tobacco in any form should be forbidden, whether the child smokes, snuffs, or chews it. A child who has smoked for a fairly brief period has a much easier time stopping than the person who has had the habit for years.

Parents must be clear on this point and need to set an example by quitting themselves if they are smokers. It's ridiculous for parents to go on smoking while sermonizing to their children on the dangers of tobacco use. Head to Chapter 11 for details on kicking a smoking habit.

✔ **Quitting illegal drugs:** Illegal drugs like amphetamines and cocaine cause high blood pressure.

✔ **Reducing salt:** Salt reduction, which I discuss in Chapter 10, is key to lowering blood pressure. The child can discover how to enjoy the taste of foods that aren't salty, and this essential step promotes lifelong control of salt intake. Managing salt at this stage may even prevent high blood pressure as the child becomes an adult.

Diets that raise the potassium can lower the blood pressure even more. Foods especially high in potassium include bananas, beet greens, broccoli, carrots, cauliflower, lettuce, oranges, spinach, and tomatoes.

The points in the preceding list can help lower blood pressure, but the child may need medication as well. I discuss medication later in this chapter.

If the child has uncomplicated high blood pressure with no kidney or heart damage, the goal of treatment is less than the 95th percentile for his sex, age, and height. If diabetes or kidney or heart damage is present, the goal is less than the 90th percentile. More info on percentiles and their ranges are in the earlier section "Interpreting the Results of the Measurement."

Advising Your Child about Strenuous Exercise

Many children want to engage in strenuous exercise and sports and don't want high blood pressure or any other abnormality to prevent them from doing so. In the absence of *severe high blood pressure* or damage to the eyes, kidneys, or heart, children can do just about any form of physical exercise they desire. Not taking height into consideration, these are the general ranges for severe high blood pressure:

- ✔ Ages 6 through 9: Greater than 129/85 mm Hg

- ✔ Ages 10 through 12: Greater than 133/89 mm Hg

- ✔ Ages 13 through 15: Greater than 143/91 mm Hg

- ✔ Ages 16 through 18: Greater than 149/97 mm Hg

When severe high blood pressure is present, children shouldn't participate in competitive sports or sports that require a great deal of physical exertion over a short period of time (like bodybuilding, rowing, and boxing). They may participate in these sports when blood pressure is under control and there is no evidence of damage to their eyes, kidneys, or heart. Less strenuous activities such as jogging are permissible.

If high blood pressure and a disease of the heart or the blood vessels are present, the severity of the heart or blood vessel disease determines the child's level of exercise. If your child has heart disease, talk to your child's doctor to come up with an appropriate exercise plan.

All athletes, but especially the athlete with high blood pressure, should avoid cocaine, tobacco, alcohol, and excessive salt — in addition to the drugs that supposedly build up the muscles or energy (like growth hormones). *Note:* Some of the mainstays in the treatment of high blood pressure, especially diuretics and beta blockers, may be illegal for athletes in particular sports. These athletes need to use other medications that aren't banned by their sport.

The bottom line is that high blood pressure doesn't shut the door to athletic performance, but physical activity must be pursued wisely, especially when the blood pressure is severe or damage to the eyes, kidneys, or heart occurs.

Using Drug Therapy

The following conditions indicate the need for drug treatment in children with high blood pressure:

- ✔ Damage to target organs like the heart and kidneys

- ✔ Diabetes

- ✔ Secondary high blood pressure

- ✔ Symptoms such as headache, nosebleeds, or dizziness

- ✔ Continued high blood pressure despite weight loss, salt reduction, and exercise

The drug treatment for children with high blood pressure is similar to the treatment of adults, though at lower doses (see Chapter 13):

- ✔ Treat mild high blood pressure with a low-dose diuretic, equivalent to 12.5 mg of hydrochlorothiazide.
- ✔ If a second drug is necessary, the most common choice is a beta blocker.
- ✔ If the combination of a diuretic and a beta blocker doesn't control blood pressure, then an ACE inhibitor, an angiotensin II receptor blocker, or a calcium channel blocker can be added. These have been recently shown to be safe in children.

Just as adults with diabetes do better with ACE inhibitors, children with diabetes should be given this drug first.

If possible, a single medication is always best because children are reluctant to take one pill a day, much less two pills two or three times a day.

Frequent monitoring is important prior to starting drug treatment and while the child is taking the drug to check the effect of the drug and to be sure the child is actually taking the medication. A parent can do this at home, checking the blood pressure every few days. After they're forced to take a pill every day, most children gladly start to make lifestyle changes such as a reduction in food intake, a reduction in salt, or an increase in exercise. Each of these changes may result in an elimination of the pill.

Stopping blood pressure medication after a year or so of successful blood pressure control is worthwhile to determine whether medication can be permanently discontinued. Be sure you work with your child's doctor on this plan!

No one knows the long-term effects of medications for high blood pressure on the growth and development of children. However, researchers are working on these questions as you read this, so we may have some answers soon.

Chapter 16

Treating High Blood Pressure in Women

*P*roviding medical care to a pregnant woman (so far, I haven't helped any pregnant men) is one of a physician's more gratifying activities. You start out with a happy woman and end up with a thrilled woman and a healthy new life — that is, most of the time. On occasion, I have run into patients who have medical problems like high blood pressure associated with a pregnancy.

The following factors apply to high blood pressure and pregnancies:

✔ May appear before or during the pregnancy and may be temporary or permanent

✔ Occurs in about 10 percent of first pregnancies and 8 percent of all pregnancies

✔ Is more common in women who previously used oral contraceptives

Most of the time, high blood pressure management during pregnancy is simple and straightforward. Only rarely does a pregnant woman suddenly develop signs and symptoms around the middle of the pregnancy that put her and her growing fetus at risk for sickness and even death. Fortunately, this complication (*preeclampsia;* I discuss it later in this chapter) has become unusual, but it still happens. For this reason, you need to be aware of it if you're the pregnant woman, the future father, or a caring friend or relative.

In this chapter, you discover the different ways that high blood pressure develops during pregnancy, its various causes, and the necessary treatments. I hope you come away from this chapter with a greater appreciation for the miracle of birth and a better understanding of blood pressure management when high blood pressure complicates this miracle.

Understanding How a Woman's Blood Pressure Responds to Pregnancy

Blood pressure isn't the same during a pregnancy as before the pregnancy. The pregnant woman's body goes through many changes to provide the best possible environment for the growing fetus. The mother-to-be must sustain the placenta, the umbilical cord (the connection between the mother and the fetus), and the fetus itself with nutrition and fluid. To do this, the expectant mother's blood vessels widen, and the volume of water and salt increases in her body. She gains about 8 liters (2 gallons) of water.

The opening of blood vessels normally causes the blood pressure to fall during the first six months of the pregnancy. (A woman with pre-existing high blood pressure may even be able to stop high blood pressure medications during pregnancy because the blood pressure may drop into the normal range.)

Pre-existing conditions, especially those related to high blood pressure, are extremely important to control during a pregnancy. Work with your doctor if

✔ **You suffer from kidney disease.** The risk of kidney failure increases significantly during pregnancy. Potential mothers should discuss with their doctor whether pregnancy is advisable.

For this reason, be sure to get a complete medical evaluation prior to becoming pregnant for any evidence of target-organ damage (damage to the organs that high blood pressure affects, especially in the heart, kidneys, and eyes). For more on target-organ damage, see Chapter 8.

✔ **You're on ACE inhibitors or angiotensin receptor blockers.** These must be stopped because they may damage the fetus. Other classes may be used prior to becoming pregnant.

✔ **You have high blood pressure before you become pregnant.** Have your doctor check your blood pressure after you become pregnant to see whether you can reduce or stop blood pressure medication.

✔ **You have high blood pressure before your pregnancy and are able to stop your medications for the first six months.** I suggest you stay off the medications for the rest of the pregnancy, even if your blood pressure rises — so long as you have no eye, kidney, or heart damage. *Note:* You may be able to stay off the meds as you breast-feed as well.

Hormones that work their magic during pregnancy

During pregnancy, the increased production of various hormones fosters fetal growth and sustains and prepares the mother-to-be for delivery and breast-feeding.

✔ An increase in *estrogen* may be responsible for some of the increased blood flow.

✔ *Progesterone* increases and helps to maintain the placenta; it also prevents the uterus from contracting.

✔ *Prolactin* increases during pregnancy in preparation for breast-feeding.

✔ *Relaxin,* a recently discovered hormone from the placenta, helps to open blood vessels.

✔ The production of *renin* (an enzyme made by the kidney when it detects a fall in blood pressure) increases (see Chapter 4) during pregnancy. The placenta is also a source of renin.

Recognizing What Causes High Blood Pressure during Pregnancy

Several factors cause high blood pressure during pregnancy. Differentiating between high blood pressure that began before the pregnancy from high blood pressure that starts during the pregnancy is important because the consequences are completely different.

If you're thinking of becoming pregnant in the near future, get a blood pressure measurement and record it. Then, if your blood pressure is high during your pregnancy, you and your doctor will know whether the reading is new or has been at that level for awhile.

Chronic high blood pressure

A woman with chronic high blood pressure has a blood pressure of more than 140/90 mm Hg on repeated occasions, and it's present before pregnancy or recognized before the 20th week of the pregnancy. Because many women haven't had their blood pressure measured before a pregnancy and because blood pressure falls normally during the first six months of a pregnancy, chronic high blood pressure may go unnoticed until the final three months of the pregnancy.

As I note in the previous section, a woman with chronic high blood pressure may be able to stop medication until the baby is born. There is no evidence that the outcome of the pregnancy improves if the mother's blood pressure is treated for the short duration of a pregnancy. However, if the diastolic blood pressure is above 100 mm Hg or the mother's heart or kidneys are damaged, she should continue the medication.

The favorite medication for high blood pressure during pregnancy is *methyl-dopa* (see Chapter 13) because it's effective and safe for both the mother and the growing fetus. If the woman is already on a diuretic (see Chapter 13), she can continue it, but she should not *start* taking it during the pregnancy because it tends to lower the blood volume — which needs to be greater during a pregnancy. If methyldopa is ineffective, *labetalol* is another drug that has been successful.

If you're pregnant and have high blood pressure, become familiar with the drugs in Chapter 13. Do not take any of the *angiotensin-converting enzyme (ACE) inhibitors,* the *angiotensin II receptor blockers,* or the *direct renin inhibitors* because they all endanger the fetus. They must be stopped as soon as a woman becomes pregnant, preferably before pregnancy.

A woman who begins a pregnancy with a diagnosis of chronic high blood pressure should not do strenuous exercise during the pregnancy. The risk to the fetal blood supply is too great.

Chronic high blood pressure poses increased risks to the mother and the fetus, and these risks are even more dangerous in African American women and women with diastolic blood pressure over 110 mm Hg. The main risks are

- ✔ Developing preeclampsia (see the following section)
- ✔ Disease such as retarded growth and death for the fetus

  This must be monitored with monthly ultrasound studies.

- ✔ Significant worsening of the mother's kidney function if kidney disease is present

Preeclampsia

Preeclampsia is high blood pressure associated with symptoms such as headache, weight gain, blurred vision, swelling, and abdominal pain along with more than 300 milligrams of protein in your urine in a 24-hour period. If unchecked, preeclampsia can lead to seizures. Dangerous for both the fetus and the mother, preeclampsia begins after the 20th week of the pregnancy, but delivering the baby and the placenta usually cures it.

Although its cause is unknown, preeclampsia occurs in roughly 5 percent of all pregnancies in most advanced nations but in greater numbers in more disadvantaged countries. You're at higher risk of developing preeclampsia if you are

- ✔ Having your first baby (especially if you're older than 40 or younger than 19) or this is your first baby with a new partner
- ✔ Carrying twins

You're also at higher risk of developing preeclampsia if you have

- ✔ High blood pressure already
- ✔ Diabetes with diabetic complications such as eye disease, kidney disease, or nerve disease (see *Diabetes For Dummies* by yours truly [Wiley])
- ✔ Any pre-existing kidney disease before becoming pregnant
- ✔ Had preeclampsia in a previous pregnancy
- ✔ A mother with preeclampsia

In the following sections, I explain how to try to prevent preeclampsia, diagnose it, and treat a worsening case. I also discuss what to do when preeclampsia turns into *eclampsia* (severe narrowing of the blood vessels in the mother's brain).

Attempting to prevent preeclampsia

At this time, preeclampsia can't be prevented, and several treatments that were tried in the past haven't worked. For these reasons, the mother-to-be needs to remain in the best health possible in case preeclampsia develops.

To improve the prospects for the pregnancy, the mother-to-be needs to eliminate anything that harms the fetus or the mother. In that respect, both tobacco and alcohol must be stopped at the beginning of a pregnancy if not before. (See Chapter 11 for more on tobacco and alcohol use.)

An important factor in the development of preeclampsia is the production of the chemicals that constrict arteries enough to raise blood pressure and inhibit the chemicals that open arteries. Researchers originally thought that aspirin would be useful because it can inhibit the constricting chemicals. But studies have not shown aspirin to be effective in decreasing the number of cases of preeclampsia.

Calcium was also suggested as a possible prevention because it seems to reduce the occurrence of preeclampsia, but it has not proved to be helpful either. Calcium doesn't reduce the cases of preeclampsia or delay the beginning of the condition.

Diagnosing preeclampsia

Preeclampsia is usually diagnosed when the following two conditions occur:

- ✔ The blood pressure rises to or above 140/90 mm Hg after the 20th week.
- ✔ The urine contains excessive levels of protein.

    Protein in the urine isn't always a result of preeclampsia. Protein loss usually accompanies swelling of the expectant mother's body, but swelling is so common during pregnancy that it's not used to diagnose preeclampsia.

There is no specific diagnostic test for preeclampsia. Usually, the expectant mother with preeclampsia experiences some or all of the following symptoms:

- ✔ Abdominal pain
- ✔ Abnormal liver enzymes in the blood
- ✔ Blurred vision
- ✔ Excessive and rapid weight gain
- ✔ Headache
- ✔ Low platelet counts in the blood resulting in abnormal clotting and bleeding
- ✔ Nausea

TIP

If your doctor only suspects that you have preeclampsia, ask her to treat you as though you do have it. Preeclampsia is one condition that should be over-diagnosed because the results can be so devastating for the mother and the fetus. Also, as in any diagnosis of high blood pressure, you should have more than one measurement of blood pressure. *Note:* Because this is a serious and dangerous disease, the measurements should be no more than a few days (or even hours) apart.

Note: Some pregnant women exhibit certain signs of preeclampsia (headache, nausea, and pain in the abdomen) but don't have high blood pressure. This is the *HELLP syndrome,* an acronym for *hemolytic anemia, elevated liver enzymes,* and *low platelets,* a serious condition that generally disappears after delivery of the baby. Some doctors consider it a variant of preeclampsia; the cause is not known and the only treatment is delivery of the baby.

Worsening preeclampsia

As preeclampsia worsens, some or all of its signs and symptoms become more severe and new symptoms develop. Headaches become more persistent and painful, restlessness increases, and pain over the stomach worsens. Among the new findings are

- ✔ Development of anemia (low red blood cell count) because of *hemolysis* (the breaking up of red blood cells)
- ✔ Increasing kidney failure
- ✔ Increasing levels of uric acid (which normally falls in early pregnancy) in the blood
- ✔ Increased blood clotting demonstrated in blood tests
- ✔ Heart failure in the mother
- ✔ Any suggestion of a rupture of the placenta with bleeding

✔ Abnormal nonstress test of the fetus

The nonstress test consists of measuring the rate of the fetal heart when it moves. A heart rate that doesn't increase with fetal movement is abnormal.

✔ Evidence of reduced fetal growth

At this point, the situation is extremely serious and treatment must be immediate. This situation must be managed in the hospital with the aid of an experienced physician.

Treating preeclampsia

One form of treatment that cures the preeclampsia is termination of the pregnancy. So when the pregnancy is at 36 weeks or longer, delivery can take place immediately. However, if the pregnancy hasn't continued to at least the 28th week, the fetus may not be mature enough to survive. Therefore, if the preeclampsia is not worsening and the mother's life is not in danger, the doctor will attempt to prolong the pregnancy as long as possible. Each extra day means a great deal for the safer delivery of the baby.

Some of the steps the doctor can take to avoid early delivery include

✔ Lowering the mother's blood pressure to between 90 and 110 mm Hg diastolic

Intravenous medications are often used for an immediate effect.

✔ Giving the mother magnesium sulfate intravenously to prevent convulsions (the complication that turns preeclampsia into eclampsia)

✔ Constant monitoring (blood pressure, the mother's weight, fetal movements, and urine protein)

✔ Establishing complete bed rest for the mother if the preeclampsia is more severe

✔ Continuing a good diet for the mother, with no reduction in salt to avoid further decreasing the blood volume of the mother

Given these steps, the mother and the fetus can avoid the complications of preeclampsia, and most mothers can avoid moving from preeclampsia to eclampsia (which I discuss in the following section).

The best route for the baby's delivery is through the vagina, which eliminates the added stress of surgery. During the delivery, the mother is given an anesthesia by way of a needle in the lower back (the epidural or spinal space) because general anesthesia can bring on increased blood pressure as a breathing tube is inserted and removed.

Probable causes of preeclampsia

Although researchers don't know the cause of preeclampsia, they do know that one of the initiating events is the failure of tissue from the placenta to connect properly with the *spiral arteries* (blood vessels in the uterus). The result is that the fetus doesn't receive sufficient nutrition. This poor connection has a greater tendency to occur in a twin pregnancy that's complicated by *hydatidiform moles* (fluid-filled cysts that replace the placenta and fetus), diabetes, and a prior history of high blood pressure.

When the placenta detects inadequate blood supply to the fetus, it begins to produce more of a hormone that raises blood pressure and less of a hormone that lowers blood pressure. One result of this hormone imbalance is a rise in blood pressure. ***Note:*** Other chemical factors cause the additional problems of increased clotting and liver damage.

Another suspected contribution to the development of preeclampsia is the body's immune system. In a normal pregnancy, the mother's immune system doesn't reject the tissue of the fetus (which is *foreign* to the mother and would be rejected under other circumstances). But in preeclampsia, the mother's immune system rejects the fetal tissue to some extent. Interestingly, the incidence of preeclampsia is lower when the mother-to-be has had prolonged sexual contact with the father prior to the pregnancy; her body has had time to become accustomed to his tissues, the same foreign tissue that the fetus now contains.

Preeclampsia is probably hereditary because it occurs more often in the daughters of mothers who had it.

After the baby is delivered, the mother's abnormalities usually disappear in a few days or weeks unless the injury to certain organs like the kidneys has been severe. In this case, organ damage may be permanent. (Testing over time can determine the extent.) If organ damage isn't permanent, the risk of preeclampsia in future pregnancies is low — though higher than if the condition hadn't occurred. In addition, the mother doesn't usually suffer from permanent high blood pressure.

Dealing with eclampsia

If the mother-to-be is diagnosed with preeclampsia and has convulsions, the condition moves to *eclampsia*. Fortunately, it occurs rarely — about once in every 2,000 pregnancies — but it can threaten the life of the mother and the fetus.

Eclampsia results from severe narrowing of the blood vessels in the brain of the mother, which then diminishes the supply of nutrients to the brain cells. Convulsions usually take place before the baby is delivered, but they can occur after delivery, too. High blood pressure isn't always present; one out of five patients has a blood pressure of less than 140/90 mm Hg just before convulsing.

The convulsions don't always take place conveniently in a hospital setting. If they occur at home, it's essential to know how to deal with them:

1. **Turn the woman on her side to improve blood flow to the placenta and to help prevent her stomach contents from moving into the lungs.**

2. **Insert a padded stick into her mouth to prevent her from biting her tongue.**

3. **Call 9-1-1 for emergency help and transportation to the hospital.**

After the patient arrives in the hospital or if the convulsions occur in the hospital:

- ✔ The doctor administers magnesium sulfate to stop the convulsions.

- ✔ If necessary, the blood pressure is controlled with medication into the vein.

- ✔ The fetus is monitored.

When everything appears to be more stable (usually within hours), the doctor delivers the baby. Although vaginal delivery is preferable, a Cesarean section is performed if time is critical.

After delivery, the mother continues on magnesium sulfate for several days until the signs of preeclampsia and eclampsia are clearly diminishing. A good indicator is when the mother's body begins excreting the large amount of extra fluid her body has accumulated.

Just as with preeclampsia, a mother who has had eclampsia

- ✔ Is likely to have normal pregnancies in the future

- ✔ Is no more likely to have high blood pressure later in life than women who've never had eclampsia

Preeclampsia on top of chronic high blood pressure

When preeclampsia complicates chronic high blood pressure during a pregnancy, the risks for the mother and the fetus are greater than the risks from either condition alone. Determining whether the chronic high blood pressure is getting worse or preeclampsia is beginning may be difficult, but a number of signs point to the onset of preeclampsia. The most useful of these signs are

- ✔ Protein in the urine when previous tests showed none

- ✔ A sudden increase in protein in the urine

✔ A sudden increase in high blood pressure that has previously been controlled

✔ A platelet count in the blood of less than 1 hundred thousand per cubic millimeter, which means a tendency to bleed easily

✔ Abnormal liver function

The treatment of preeclampsia in association with chronic high blood pressure must be even more attentive than the treatment of preeclampsia alone. The decision to end such a pregnancy is made even earlier than when high blood pressure isn't a complication.

Gestational high blood pressure

Gestational high blood pressure (associated with a pregnancy) is *transient* high blood pressure when:

✔ No preeclampsia is associated with the pregnant woman's high blood pressure

✔ The high blood pressure disappears 12 weeks after delivery

Transient high blood pressure is usually found after the middle of the pregnancy but without protein in the urine or any of the other signs or symptoms of preeclampsia. This condition isn't treated during pregnancy because it seems to cause no setback for mother or fetus.

This form of high blood pressure usually disappears a few days after delivery, but it's not entirely benign. It tends to reoccur in future pregnancies (again not causing any problem) and seems to be a marker for *essential* high blood pressure (high blood pressure for which the cause is unknown) some years later.

Dealing with High Blood Pressure after Delivery

If the mother has chronic high blood pressure, she can take three drugs to manage her high blood pressure while she breast-feeds: *methyldopa, timolol,* and *nifedipine* (check these out in Chapter 13). Although all three are excreted in breast milk, studies show that these meds do not hurt the baby in any way.

If you're breast-feeding, ask your doctor about the possibility of withholding blood pressure medications. As long as you're carefully monitored for elevations in blood pressure, this is a safe option.

Following delivery, the mother can safely add some of the useful techniques for lowering blood pressure that I discuss in Part III. In particular, a combination of salt reduction, weight loss, and exercise can speed up recovery from the stress of pregnancy and help to reduce blood pressure without the use of drugs.

Using Female Hormone Treatment in the Presence of High Blood Pressure

Women take estrogen and progesterone for two major indications: to prevent conception before menopause and to replace missing hormones after menopause. Although earlier formulations were associated with increases in blood pressure, the current treatments are only occasionally associated with an increase in blood pressure. The following sections guide you through hormone use that avoids the occurrence of high blood pressure.

Hormones for oral contraception

Just exactly how the oral contraceptives raise blood pressure is unknown. No particular factor (like weight, age, or ethnic origin) seems to predict who will have an increase in blood pressure and to what extent. In the past, most women who took oral contraceptives had a rise in blood pressure that was usually mild, rarely severe. The newer preparations of oral contraceptives contain much smaller doses of both estrogen and progesterone. Today the increase in blood pressure is less frequent, probably a result of the reduced dosage.

Women who smoke and are over age 35 are more sensitive to oral contraceptives and shouldn't take them. Although the rise in blood pressure doesn't damage most of these women, occasionally the kidneys are damaged. If concern exists about blood pressure, then the woman should discontinue the oral contraceptive, which will cause a prompt fall in her blood pressure.

If you plan to take oral contraceptives, you must stop smoking (a good idea even if you don't plan to take them!). Make sure your blood pressure is measured before you start the contraceptives and every six months while you take them. If you have a blood pressure increase of 20 mm Hg systolic or 10 mm Hg diastolic, replace the oral contraceptive with a different form of contraception.

Doctors don't usually prescribe drugs for increased blood pressure when oral contraceptives appear to be the source of the increase, but occasionally no other form of contraception is possible. In these cases, the usual treatment is lifestyle modification and, if necessary, drugs to lower blood pressure. See Chapter 13.

Hormones for estrogen replacement

Prehypertension (see Chapter 2) is extremely common among postmenopausal women. In fact, a study in the February 2007 *Circulation* showed that 40 percent of all women in the postmenopausal age range have prehypertension. Any medication that can possibly turn that condition into high blood pressure must be carefully evaluated.

Because blood pressure rises as people age, researchers were concerned that estrogen replacement therapy would make this rise worse, given estrogen's known effect as part of the oral contraceptives. However, replacement therapy uses much lower doses of estrogens than oral contraceptives, and that lower dose may actually lower blood pressure. One form that has been especially useful in lowering blood pressure is *transdermal estrogen* (estrogen given as a patch or gel applied to the skin).

Estrogen replacement isn't a treatment for high blood pressure, but because it tends to lower blood pressure, it's safe for a postmenopausal woman with blood pressure concerns. *Note:* If a woman already has high blood pressure, estrogen therapy doesn't aggravate it.

The major concern about hormone replacement after menopause is the finding that it increases the risk of heart attacks (see Chapter 5) and brain attacks (see Chapter 7). However, a study in the April 2007 *Journal of the American Medical Association* showed that women who started hormone replacement at the beginning of menopause didn't have an increased risk compared with women who started hormone replacement several years after menopause. The bottom line is that unless your menopausal symptoms are severe, you're better off without hormone replacement.

Part V
The Part of Tens

The 5th Wave   By Rich Tennant

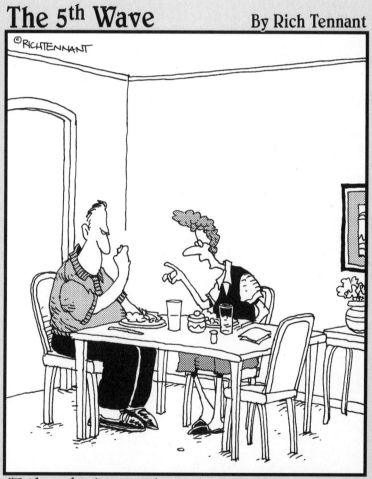

"I thought it would encourage you to reduce your sodium intake. It's a salt dispenser in the shape of a constricted artery."

In this part . . .

*I*f you want to know simple tricks to lower your blood pressure and keep it normal, you can find them in this part. In addition, I provide a list of myths about treatment so you can avoid errors in treating your high blood pressure. And finally, I give you the scoop on the latest medical discoveries about high blood pressure.

Chapter 17

Ten Simple Ways to Prevent or Reduce High Blood Pressure

*I*n this chapter, I offer ten of the many ways that you can prevent or lower high blood pressure. All of them are fairly simple. You actually know what you have to do already. Do I need to tell you to stop smoking and drinking? Do mice play baseball?

The trick is to adopt at least two of the ideas in this chapter. If you succeed at both, you're well on your way to reducing your blood pressure to an agreeable level. Most importantly, don't fall back into old bad habits! Now's the time to make a permanent change. In the immortal words of Shakespeare in *Henry IV,* "Strike now, or else the iron cools."

If you're determined to prevent or lower high blood pressure, you have to pay your DEWS. Follow the DASH diet, Exercise, lose Weight, and reduce Salt.

Making Sure You Have High Blood Pressure

You may save yourself a lifetime of taking unnecessary drugs by simply making sure your blood pressure is *truly* elevated, so step one is to be certain it's *persistently* elevated.

Make sure your doctor is measuring your blood pressure properly (see Chapter 2) because numerous aspects can affect its accuracy:

  ✔ Wrong size blood pressure cuff

  ✔ Wrong arm placement

✔ Not being relaxed before the measurement

✔ Speaking during the measurement

In addition, make sure you don't have *white coat high blood pressure* (blood pressure that's high only in the doctor's office when you may be nervous). A good home blood pressure device can check for this possibility. (See Chapter 2 for a whole section on home monitoring.)

Pharmacy measurement devices are notorious for their high error rate. Make sure any device you rely on is properly maintained.

Elevated blood pressure doesn't necessarily persist, especially when you make lifestyle changes or had temporary reasons for an elevation. If you're already on medication, ask your doctor whether you can lower the dose or even stop — if it's safe — after a year or more.

Determining Whether You Have Secondary High Blood Pressure

About 5 percent of high blood pressure cases have a definite, treatable cause, so the diagnosis is then *secondary high blood pressure.* If your doctor can discover the cause and then cure it (especially early on), it can eliminate your high blood pressure (and the need for medication) and perhaps prevent other damage to your body.

Clues that suggest secondary high blood pressure include the following:

✔ High blood pressure that develops suddenly in childhood or past the age of 50

✔ The body's resistance to drug treatment

✔ Changes in the patient's body shape and pigmentation

✔ Attacks of coldness and pallor along with the high blood pressure

✔ No family history of high blood pressure (high blood pressure tends to run in families)

When a doctor suspects secondary high blood pressure, he should test for a specific diagnosis (see Chapter 4). Shooting at every possible diagnosis is wasteful and usually unproductive.

Unfortunately, kidney damage is frequently the cause of secondary high blood pressure. The kidney can't be repaired, but the doctor can prescribe specific blood pressure drugs that are better for the kidneys.

Adopting the DASH Diet

A study published in the *New England Journal of Medicine* (April 1997) introduced the *Dietary Approach to Stop Hypertension* (DASH) diet. This diet (see details in Chapter 9) may be the best treatment of high blood pressure in decades.

The DASH diet requires you to eat a mix of grains, fruits, and vegetables and low-fat or nonfat dairy products while you reduce the intake of high-fat dairy products, meats, fats, and sweets. The diet also encourages a weekly amount of nuts and seeds.

One of the best features is that the recommended foods are the ones you eat each day — no special supplements, vitamins, or minerals; no daily visits to group therapy. In addition:

- ✔ You don't need to take a drug that reduces your appetite because you're not reducing your kilocalories.
- ✔ You aren't left feeling hungry.
- ✔ You don't even have to exercise to lower your pressure.
- ✔ You don't miss the meat and dairy products because you're still getting them — just not so many.
- ✔ DASH contains foods that you (rather than a food manufacturer) usually prepare.
- ✔ Many people find that they can follow this diet permanently.

You don't even have to change your diet all at once. Start reducing the meat and dairy and substituting some grains. Add more vegetables; use fruits for dessert instead of cookies, cake, or ice cream. Before you know it, you'll be DASHing.

Combining DASH (where salt reduction takes place automatically) with a further reduction in salt can double the lowering effects on your high blood pressure. Don't add salt to food, and try to keep your salt intake under 1,500 milligrams every day (see the later section for more info).

 After you read Chapter 9, consider the services of a knowledgeable dietitian (make sure she's well versed in the requirements of DASH), and check out this excellent Web site: www.nhlbi.nih.gov/hbp/prevent/h_eating/h_eating.htm.

Losing Weight by Reducing Kilocalorie Intake

A great way to lower your blood pressure is to lose weight by reducing the number of kilocalories you eat. (See Chapter 9 to determine your weight loss and daily caloric needs.) If you're overweight or obese with high blood pressure, you may want to really hit the jackpot: Combine the DASH diet (see the previous section) with low salt and weight loss. First, determine your *body mass index* or *BMI*. (Again, Chapter 9 walks you through this.) If your BMI is 25 to 29.9, you're *overweight;* if it's 30 or above, you're *obese.* In terms of high blood pressure risks, you're not out of the woods at 24.5; you're better off with a BMI of 23.5.

The key term for reducing kilocalories is *substitution.* Simply substitute a low-calorie food for a higher-calorie food. For example, rather than eating a handful of cookies, eat an apple to save about 100 kilocalories.

Some of the best substitutions include:

- ✔ Snacking on fruits and vegetables instead of chips and soft drinks
- ✔ Eating skinless, white-meat chicken instead of dark-meat chicken with skin
- ✔ Choosing nonfat or low-fat dairy products in place of high-fat cheeses
- ✔ Choosing prepared foods that have fewer kilocalories instead of less fat

Use the Nutrition Facts label on all prepared foods to find out the fat, kilocalories, and salt per portion. The government's gone to so much trouble getting food producers to label their foods. Give that label a close look.

Many kilocalories can be added or cut back during food preparation. Preferable foods are broiled, cooked in their own juices, poached, grilled, blackened, or baked. Avoid foods that are battered and fried or made in a butter, cream, plum, cheese, or sweet-and-sour sauce.

The key to maintaining your weight loss is the level of your motivation. If joining a weight-loss group helps keep you motivated, do it. (Every study I've seen shows the value of continuing to participate on a regular basis, so stay with it!)

Reducing Salt in Your Diet

The easiest way to bring down your high blood pressure is to take as much salt out of your diet as possible. Don't worry that you won't get enough. You need only 500 milligrams (⅛ teaspoon) each day, which you can achieve if you eat only natural foods. But because most Americans consume 5,000 milligrams (3 teaspoons) each day, 1,500 milligrams (1 teaspoon) a day is more realistic.

Prepared foods account for 75 percent of the salt in your diet, so consider these suggestions:

- ✔ Cut back on the number of prepared foods you buy (for example, prepared soups and crackers).

- ✔ Consult the Nutrition Facts label to check the amount of salt in each portion. Even if the salt content appears low, eating too many portions can put your salt level over the top.

- ✔ Cut back on chips and crackers.

    Substitute low-salt chips or, even better, fresh fruit or raw vegetables for snacks high in salt.

Another 10 percent of the salt that you eat is naturally in food, but the final 15 percent is from the saltshaker. Try keeping the saltshaker off the table.

Saltaholics (people who insist on lots of salt) are missing all kinds of great tastes. If you fall into this category, try preparing your food with half the usual amount of salt — the natural tastes may pleasantly surprise you.

If you still need more flavor, though, try adding herbs and spices. For canned vegetables, try washing out much of the salt with plain water and then add herbs and spices.

Monitoring the amount of salt in your food is rather difficult when you eat out. Chefs tend to add salt liberally. But you can ask for the food to be prepared with little or no salt or choose a restaurant that offers low-salt items on the menu. Your local chapter of the American Heart Association may list local restaurants that serve low-salt food.

You may be able to eliminate a high-blood-pressure drug by significantly reducing your salt intake. Tell me that's not a bargain! For more about curbing salt in your diet, head to Chapter 10.

Giving Up Tobacco and Excess Alcohol

Both tobacco and alcohol raise blood pressure, but that's just the tip of the iceberg for these addicting substances. Consider these facts:

- ✔ Because of the nicotine, tobacco in any form (smoked, chewed, or snuffed) raises blood pressure. About 33 percent of the people with high blood pressure are smokers.

    Any regular exposure to tobacco is dangerous. If you smoke, you're damaging your own health *and* compromising the health of your loved ones. Spouses and children of smokers have a much higher rate of lung disease, asthma, and cancer than the spouses and children of nonsmokers. That's no way to treat someone you love.

✔ Excessive amounts of alcohol (more than two glasses of wine for a man or one glass for a woman every night) raise blood pressure. In addition, three or four glasses add many kilocalories (375 to 500) to your daily total, and your relaxed state from that much alcohol doesn't lend itself to careful eating and salt restriction. (Recent studies seem to indicate that a glass or two of red wine protects your heart from heart disease. However, too much of a good thing is bad for you.)

Smoking and drinking often go hand in hand. You may do better to concentrate on stopping one of them and, therefore, eliminating many of the situations where you do the other. Check Chapter 11 for advice on how to stop smoking and drinking.

Starting an Exercise Program

If you don't want to lose weight or curb your salt intake (although I strongly advise both), you can still lower your blood pressure with exercise. But you have to choose an exercise program that you can stick to. When the plan requires much more than the person's prepared to do on a long-term basis, the regimen doesn't last.

Make sure you're in good enough health to start your exercise program by visiting your doctor for a checkup.

A regular walking or jogging program works best for most people (check Chapter 12 for a complete program and its benefits). Design your program to start slowly for short distances and build up to 45 minutes of exercise three or four times a week. You don't have to join a club to do it.

Another form of exercise that you may want to add is weight lifting. Start off lifting a light weight and work your way up slowly. *Note:* If you have very high blood pressure (greater than 180/110 mm Hg), weight lifting isn't a good idea. However, people at lower levels can benefit from it.

Exercise doesn't just lower blood pressure. It increases self-esteem, improves balance, fights depression, enhances memory, and generally makes you very aware that life is worth living.

Enhancing Your Treatment with Mind-Body Techniques

Some Eastern disciplines lower blood pressure. I'm not suggesting that you ignore Western medicine and follow the paths of the East; however, mind-body techniques such as yoga, meditation, and hypnosis can enhance your current course of treatment. If you can lower your blood pressure just a few millimeters (and reap other benefits at the same time — like a more focused and serene mind), it's worthwhile. (See Chapter 12 for more information on mind-body techniques.)

The following mind-body techniques should be an *addition* to the salt reduction, weight loss, and exercise that you do already, not a substitute. On the other hand, effective use of these techniques *may* eventually replace the role of medications in your treatment. After you become proficient, you can think about stopping a blood pressure medication ***Note:*** Never stop taking doctor-prescribed medications on your own. Work with your doctor every step of the way.

- ✔ **Yoga:** This technique emphasizes postures and proper breathing. People coming out of a yoga class almost always express how relaxed and warm they feel. When their blood pressure is taken, it's usually lower than before the class.

- ✔ **Meditation:** This technique calms the mind by concentrating on an object, a sound, a word, or the breath. Just 20 minutes twice each day seems to be enough to provide a day's worth of blood pressure control. For people against exercise in any form, this blood-pressure-lowering technique may be just right.

- ✔ **Hypnosis:** By the process of self-suggestion, you can tell yourself to be calm and to lower your stress level and your blood pressure. Hypnotism isn't a game, but a useful tool that may be your answer to controlling your blood pressure.

- ✔ **Biofeedback:** This technique uses a *biofeedback machine* to detect a person's internal bodily functions (such as high blood pressure) in order to alter a function. Because biofeedback requires equipment, it may be a little less desirable than the other methods. But if you can't engage in the other mind-body techniques, then this may be the solution for you.

One of my favorite techniques is humor therapy. (See Chapter 8 for more on this.) If you walk into a room where everyone's laughing for no apparent reason, you may have found your way into a humor club. Imagine! They don't even need a source of humor. They just go ahead and laugh, regardless of the consequences, which may include a fall in blood pressure. Laughter can also reduce stress hormones and improve immune function. Try it, you'll like it.

Using Drugs to Lower Blood Pressure

Have you tried every technique short of medication but your blood pressure still measures more than 140/90 mm Hg? If you haven't received the desired result, you need to discuss medication options with your doctor.

More than 60 different medications are available for lowering blood pressure, so you're sure to find the right drug or combination of drugs for your needs. (For more information on blood-pressure-lowering drugs, see Chapter 13.) Despite so many options, most people use the same three types, which also happen to be the least expensive and most familiar to doctors:

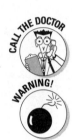

1. **Most doctors start their patients with a *diuretic*** (a medication that lowers blood pressure by forcing the body to rid itself of salt and water through the kidneys into the urine). *Hydrochlorothiazide* is available as a generic drug, and the 12.5 dosage is most effective for lowering blood pressure and prolonging life.

   With a little bit of luck, that prescription may be all you need. If you're already on a bigger dose, see whether your doctor will reduce it while monitoring your blood pressure. (He may be surprised, but you won't be because you've read this book!)

2. **Ask your doctor about adding a *beta blocker*** (a medication that blocks pressure-raising substances in the body) if the diuretic doesn't do the job or you want to get your blood pressure even lower because you're diabetic. *Propranolol* is probably the best and has proven itself for decades.

   Beta blockers can cause fatigue and reduce exercise tolerance, so they aren't a good choice for people who exercise strenuously.

   Your doctor may also prescribe a *calcium channel blocking agent* (a medication that widens blood vessels) if diuretics and beta blockers don't completely control your high blood pressure. By themselves, these blocking agents aren't as effective as diuretics or beta blockers — especially if heart failure is present or a heart attack has already occurred — but with the other meds, they may do the job.

   If your doctor suggests taking a calcium channel blocker, ask whether *nifedipine* extended-release tablets may work for you. They're an inexpensive, generic pill that you take once a day.

3. **Your doctor may decide to add a drug from the *angiotensin-converting enzyme (ACE) inhibitors* class or the similar class *angiotensin II receptor blockers* to the diuretic and the beta blocker for a three-drug combination.** For some people, especially diabetics with kidney disease, ACE inhibitors and angiotensin II receptor blockers are the treatment of choice because they lower blood pressure *and* protect the kidneys.

   Of the many drugs in these classes, *enalapril* or *lisinopril* are once-a-day and inexpensive. *Note:* Don't take these two types of drugs during a pregnancy or while breast-feeding — they're not good for the baby.

I thoroughly discuss many other drugs in Chapter 13, but, with the possible exception of *methyldopa* for pregnant women with high blood pressure, these other drugs have limited use for controlling high blood pressure.

When a patient doesn't take the prescription pills, it's called *noncompliance* — a major crime if ever there was one — and it doesn't do much for your blood pressure either!

Controlling blood pressure can prevent heart attacks, brain attacks, and kidney damage, and yet only 12.5 million of the 50 million people with high blood pressure in the United States have theirs under control. It's time to improve that statistic one patient at a time — starting with you or your loved one.

Avoiding Drugs That Raise Blood Pressure

Plenty of drugs on the market *raise* blood pressure on their own or *block* the action of a drug that lowers blood pressure. If you can avoid them, do so. (Check back to Chapter 13 for more in-depth discussions on these meds.)

Some drugs may raise blood pressure in only one person — you! Check with your doctor and monitor your blood pressure whenever you start or stop a drug. A new drug may raise the pressure or block your blood pressure drugs. Likewise, your pressure may rise when you stop taking a drug that interacted with the medication that controls your pressure.

Sometimes a patient has a problem so severe that she must take a drug that elevates her blood pressure as a side effect. In that case, the patient also has to use high blood pressure meds to overcome that effect from the essential drug. For example:

- ✔ If you have kidney disease, you may have to take *erythropoietin* to combat anemia. As much as you don't need another way for your blood pressure to elevate, erythropoietin will do it.

- ✔ *Colestipol* and *cholestyramine* lower cholesterol, but they also fight blood pressure medications. Fortunately, the choices for treating cholesterol are numerous, so you can switch if necessary.

Cold medications often contain drugs that constrict arteries and elevate blood pressure. Read the labels on all cold medication that you plan to use. Any med that can affect blood pressure has a label clearly stating that it should *not* be taken by a person who has high blood pressure. If uncertain, check with your doctor before you use it.

Diet pills that contain *phenylpropanolamine,* which is similar to *amphetamine,* raise blood pressure. Do not use these drugs if you have high blood pressure already!

Prescription drugs that may raise blood pressure include the following:

- ✔ Steroids like *cortisone* or *prednisone*
- ✔ Several antidepressant drugs
  - *Trimipramine* and *venlafaxine* in particular cause sustained increases in blood pressure.
  - Antidepressant drugs from the *monoamine oxidase inhibitors* class raise blood pressure by preventing the breakdown of *epinephrine.* Drugs in this class include *phenylzine* and *tranylcypromine.*
- ✔ Nonsteroidal anti-inflammatory agents

  The worst offenders are *indomethacin, naprosyn,* and *ibuprofen,* especially in large doses.

Oral contraceptives used to contain high amounts of *estrogen,* which made them notorious for raising blood pressure. The newer preparations with less estrogen are much better, but your blood pressure should be checked before you start and monitored after you're on them. ***Note:*** The much smaller dose of estrogen for menopause may actually lower blood pressure.

Antacids that contain an abundance of salt don't help your blood pressure. Check the label! If you're taking 900 milligrams of salt each time your stomach aches, you aren't doing your blood pressure any favors. Plenty of good choices are available like calcium- and magnesium-containing antacids.

Illegal drugs like cocaine that raise blood pressure shouldn't be taken in the first place, much less by a person who has high blood pressure.

Chapter 18

Ten (Or So) Myths about High Blood Pressure

In This Chapter

▶ Investigating misunderstandings about high blood pressure

▶ Discovering the realities of high blood pressure

*P*eople are likely to believe myths when they don't understand a subject. And those myths often provide a justification for a certain action or inaction. But I hope this chapter clears up any of your misunderstandings so you can take the actions I describe in Part III and gain complete control of your blood pressure.

Myths about high blood pressure are numerous, so selecting only ten (or so) is difficult. I tried to pick out the ones that have the most impact on your high blood pressure.

High Blood Pressure Is an Inevitable Result of Aging

One of the risk factors usually listed for high blood pressure is aging. But does aging *cause* the increase or is something else going on? In Chapter 3, I point out two populations where high blood pressure is either non-existent or extremely rare: tribes in the Amazon, who are isolated from modern civilization; and rural populations in Latin and South America, China, and Africa. These populations demonstrate that high blood pressure is not inevitable, even with aging.

A fraction of the elderly population does not have high blood pressure. However, the remaining numbers that do have high blood pressure tend to have several other factors in common:

- ✔ They're overweight or obese.
- ✔ They're sedentary, doing little or no manual labor.

✔ They eat a diet deficient in fruits and vegetables.

✔ They take in too much salt.

Each of these factors can lead to high blood pressure, even in younger individuals.

The one change that occurs with age that may lead to high blood pressure is a gradual loss of kidney function. However, this loss may be related to the factors in the previous list rather than aging itself.

You *can* prevent high blood pressure by adopting a healthy lifestyle at a young age and sticking to it. The result is not just a longer life but also a higher-quality life. See Part III for the lifestyle changes you can make to prevent (or reduce) high blood pressure.

The Treatment Is Worse Than the Disease

The consequences of untreated high blood pressure at any age are far greater than the side effects of medication or the inconveniences of lifestyle changes. For example, when you use nondrug treatments like lowering your salt and caffeine and exercising regularly, your blood pressure responds. (See Chapters 8 through 12 for more ways that you can adjust your lifestyle to lower your blood pressure.) And many nondrug treatments provide all kinds of other benefits. As far as I know, you can't get the peacefulness that comes from exercising, yoga, and meditation in any blood pressure medicine on the market!

But if your doctor determines that your blood pressure needs medication, don't have a crisis. Sure, they have side effects that you'd prefer not to have, but there aren't many worse than heart attacks, brain attacks, and kidney failure — all side effects of untreated high blood pressure.

Side effects from blood pressure meds can be overcome in several ways:

✔ Ask your doctor whether you can lower your dose while monitoring your blood pressure.

✔ If side effects are severe, ask your doctor to prescribe two different medications at lower doses to avoid the side effects of either one.

✔ If you're fatigued, ask your doctor to check your potassium. If it's low, he can add a potassium-sparing agent (see Chapter 13).

✔ If you perform some work that requires high mental alertness (like running heavy equipment or driving a car), let your doctor know. Blood pressure drugs that cause sleepiness probably aren't for you. Work with your doctor to determine the combination of lifestyle changes and medications that's right for you.

- ✔ If you're a competitive athlete, the beta blockers are probably a poor choice because they prevent your body from changing its heart rate and other parameters that are necessary for vigorous activity.

- ✔ Certain drugs *(angiotensin-converting enzyme inhibitors)* are especially helpful under special circumstances like diabetic kidney disease, but they cause side effects. Rather than losing the great benefits of these drugs, ask your doctor whether you can switch. For example, if cough is your problem, switch to an *angiotensin II receptor blocker.*

You Must Restrict Your Life Because You Have High Blood Pressure

Although high blood pressure is a serious condition that must be managed with lifestyle change and drugs if necessary, restricting your life (avoiding strenuous exercise or never eating out) isn't reasonable. The side effects of blood pressure drugs should not keep you from living a normal life.

If you have uncomplicated high blood pressure, your quality of life should be about the same as a person's with normal blood pressure. In fact, that quality can even improve because you're taking better care of your body. For example, limiting salt and kilocalories aren't so much restrictions as opportunities to enhance the quality of your life. You have a chance to taste some amazing foods that were hidden behind the strong taste of salt, and you're feeling better, more attractive, and healthier because you're restricting kilocalories and losing some weight.

People who must take a drug that makes them sleepy can't work in a profession that requires maximum alertness. But that's the *only* limitation to your life due to your high blood pressure. I've never seen a person refused a job because of high blood pressure, and terminating an employee because of it is illegal.

You Need Treatment Only for a High Diastolic Blood Pressure

In the past, doctors treated only a high diastolic blood pressure, and many doctors still follow that plan. But you know better.

Both the diastolic blood pressure and the systolic blood pressure figure in the decision to lower blood pressure. (See Chapter 2 for more information about these two numbers.) And although diastolic blood pressure tends to fall with age, systolic blood pressure tends to rise. For example, studies show these two facts:

- ✔ People with high blood pressure under the age of 50 usually have *diastolic* high blood pressure, and this condition is a predictor of whether a person is likely to develop coronary atherosclerosis.

- ✔ The much larger group (people with high blood pressure over the age of 50) usually has isolated *systolic* high blood pressure, and this type of high blood pressure can predict whether a person is likely to develop coronary atherosclerosis (see Chapter 5).

If treatment were based on the diastolic blood pressure alone, very few people over 50 would receive treatment. But treating people over age 50 for high blood pressure greatly reduces the number of heart attacks and brain attacks in this age group.

Lowering the diastolic blood pressure too much in the elderly population (older than 65) is dangerous. Their diastolic blood pressure is already low, so dropping it below 65 to 70 mm Hg with blood pressure medication results in an increase of brain attacks. In these cases, accepting a systolic blood pressure greater than 140 may be necessary in order to avoid a diastolic blood pressure below 70.

High Blood Pressure Means Pills for the Rest of Your Life

I hope the large amount of information in Part III convinces you that having high blood pressure doesn't have to mean taking pills for the rest of your life. In fact, even the best pills have side effects, so avoid them if you can.

Reducing your weight can be just as effective as any pill. The same is true for exercising, following a diet like DASH, using mind-body techniques like meditation, and reducing salt intake. Simply put, combining all these lifestyle changes can reduce blood pressure — *without* side effects — better than any pill.

Pills are a last resort when lifestyle changes can't sufficiently lower the pressure. But even then, you must continue improving your lifestyle — it may allow you to stop one or all of your pills. ***Note:*** If you do have to continue your pills, remember that the damage from high blood pressure is continuous. When you lower your pressure by a few millimeters of mercury, you reduce the danger of a stroke, a heart attack, kidney and eye damage, and other complications even though the pressure remains in the *high* classification.

You Can Give Up Treatment after a Heart or Brain Attack

Keeping your blood pressure under control is more important now than ever! One of the main risk factors for a heart attack or a brain attack is a *previous* heart or brain attack, so after you recover from a heart or brain attack, you must continue your treatment. Before you leave the hospital, plan to make the changes that can bring your blood pressure under control:

- ✔ Stop smoking

- ✔ Follow a low-salt DASH diet

- ✔ Start a lifelong exercise program (after your doctor has given the *all clear*)

- ✔ Reduce your alcohol intake if it's excessive

I describe all these changes in Part III.

The changes that help you control your high blood pressure can also help your diabetes, arthritis, and heart and blood vessels.

You Can Avoid Exercise Because of High Blood Pressure

This myth provides an excuse for many people who don't want to exercise. Not only is it totally and unequivocally false, but it's also the exact opposite of the truth. Exercise lowers blood pressure.

How did this myth get started? It may have begun in a dark alley in the Kasbah (just joking). Actually, it probably began when some people with severe, uncontrolled high blood pressure and major complications of the condition did some exercise and got into trouble. For example, a person with unstable heart disease associated with high blood pressure can have a heart attack as a result of heavy exercise.

If you have heart disease or have had a heart attack or a brain attack, ask your physician what exercises you can do safely. You may have no limitations, or you may need to avoid activities that are too vigorous or require too much effort over a short period of time (like heavy weightlifting). *Note:* Many doctors are unaware of how much you should do and may say, "Take it easy." You need better advice than that; you may want to see a cardiologist or an exercise physiologist.

If your high blood pressure is under control and you have no complications, don't avoid exercise — its benefits are enormous. (See the long list of exercises in Chapter 12.) Keep these tips in mind:

- Thirty minutes of walking a day provides great benefits.

- Select an exercise that you know you'll continue.

- Consider an exercise that you can do indoors during inclement weather. (However, I recently met a young woman who runs daily. When it rains, she uses a plastic garbage bag to keep dry.)

- A good goal is exercise that you perceive as *very hard*. Some days you may want to do less.

  Don't exercise to the point that you have chest pain or can't breathe. If you do, you may want to confer with your doctor.

The old adage for physical exercise used to be, "No pain, no gain." The new one is, "Refrain, no gain."

If You Feel Fine, You Can Skip Your Blood Pressure Medications

High blood pressure is sometimes called the *silent killer* because people are often unaware that they have it. The disease can even damage the eyes, heart, kidneys, and blood vessels before symptoms appear and organs fail — and then it's too late to reverse the damage.

This lack of symptoms is the reason many people neglect to take their blood pressure medication. They may rationalize that

- They felt fine before they started taking the pills.

- The only reason they're taking the pills is because their doctor measured a high blood pressure.

- The side effects of the pills make them feel worse.

Take your blood pressure medication! (Check out Chapter 13 for full details.)The point is to lower your pressure so you can prevent complications like heart attacks and brain attacks in the future (check out Part II). These complications probably take ten years or more to develop, so the sooner you bring your blood pressure down into the normal range, the more time you have to steer clear of these risks.

If side effects from the medication are a problem, discuss the possibility of lowering the dose or switching to another medicine with your doctor.

High Blood Pressure Can't Be Controlled

If you take your medication regularly but your blood pressure doesn't come down into the acceptable range, don't give up — and definitely don't stop taking your medication! Instead, with the help of your doctor, take another look at your medication and lifestyle to see whether you can do more to control your blood pressure.

Rest assured, there is an explanation and a way to control your high blood pressure. It's up to you and your doctor to find the right solution. Here are some guidelines:

✓ **Are you sure your blood pressure is uncontrolled?** Could it be a faulty measurement? Is your blood pressure normal except when you step into the doctor's office (white coat effect; see Chapter 2 for more info)? You may have to get your own blood pressure device and check it at home.

✓ **Is your drug treatment effective?** Resistance to treatment is the inability of a combination of three meds from three different classes (one of which is a diuretic) to lower the blood pressure to less than 140/90 mm Hg. Consider these possibilities:

- Do you have low potassium as a result of too much diuretic?

- Are you an African American taking a beta blocker, which lowers blood pressure less effectively among African Americans?

- Are you taking one daily dose of a medication that doesn't last through a full 24 hours?

- Maybe you're currently treating another medical problem with medications that are interfering with the action of your blood pressure medicines.

Check with your doctor to see whether any drug interactions are blocking your blood pressure treatment.

✓ **Are you maximizing your use of lifestyle changes to squeeze every millimeter of mercury out of those procedures?** How are your answers to these questions?

- Are you reducing your salt intake?

- Have you lost some weight and kept it off? It doesn't take much — only 5 to 10 percent of your body weight — to make a big dent in your blood pressure.

- Have you tried the DASH diet, which in many cases can lower your blood pressure as much as the best blood pressure medications?

- Have you quit smoking?

- Have you reduced or stopped your intake of caffeine?

- Have you stopped drinking more than a glass or two of wine daily?

- Are you trying some of the other methods like yoga, meditation, or laughter?

Note: You can't say that your blood pressure can't be controlled until all these methods have been put to use; see Part III for details about all of them.

Discuss with your doctor the possibility that you have secondary high blood pressure (see Chapter 4). The diseases and conditions that can cause secondary high blood pressure (blocked kidney arteries or a tumor in an adrenal gland, for example) are rare but may account for the stubborn resistance of your blood pressure to treatment.

Treatment Is Limited to Nervous, Anxious People

False. A high level of nervousness and anxiety doesn't indicate that a person has or will have high blood pressure. In fact, a nervous, anxious person may have normal blood pressure, and a person who appears quite calm and peaceful may have exceedingly high blood pressure.

This myth probably developed from the short name for high blood pressure — *hypertension.* The prefix *hyper* suggests that sufferers are highly stressed, jumpy, and nervous individuals who live a life of anger and road rage and have a short fuse that's ready to blow at any moment. The suffix *tension* certainly doesn't suggest a calm, peaceful state of being.

People with high blood pressure are in every social class, doing every type of work. And although high blood pressure tends to be a disease of the overweight, it's certainly present among thin people. And people with high blood pressure aren't necessarily type-A overachievers working 14-hour days. (It would certainly make doctors' diagnostic abilities much better if they could simply pick out the people with high blood pressure, but it doesn't work that way!)

Acute stress raises the blood pressure temporarily — this is a normal response to stress and the release of hormones. However, as stress becomes *chronic* or lasts over a long period of time, the hormones no longer release at the same rate, and the blood pressure falls.

People who move from a quiet neighborhood to a big city often have an increase in blood pressure. But this change is more the result of increased salt and weight gain than stress. Similarly, a stressful job raises the blood pressure temporarily in some people, especially men, but stress alone does not cause persistent high blood pressure.

The Elderly Don't Need to Be Treated

The elderly population (I use a definition of age 65 or older) has the greatest prevalence of high blood pressure and the highest number of heart attacks and brain attacks each year. Despite this fact, some people believe it's too late or not helpful to treat high blood pressure in the elderly. But treating them can clearly prevent large numbers of these attacks! Left untreated, these people often die earlier than normal or suffer years of disability.

Nevertheless, treating the elderly is not a simple matter (that's why I devote Chapter 14 to this subject). Many of them need assistance with their medical needs and encouragement to make lifestyle changes. For example, this age group is especially sensitive to salt, which can raise blood pressure, so simply reducing the amount of salt may successfully control their blood pressure. However, because their taste sensation is reduced, they may want to add even more. The goal is to teach them to substitute herbs and spices and make other lifestyle changes before relying on drugs. (The average elderly person already takes an average of seven drugs each day!)

The elderly usually show isolated systolic high blood pressure and low diastolic pressure. As a result, doctors must take great care not to lower the diastolic blood pressure too much — no lower than 60 to 70. This age group also has diminished kidney function, even when they have no diseases. If they do need drugs for high blood pressure, the recommendation is to start low and go slow.

High Blood Pressure Is Less Dangerous in Women

The consequences of high blood pressure for women are as serious as those for men, so controlling it is just as important for women. I cover much more on this subject in Chapter 16.

Although three out of four women who have high blood pressure are aware of it, only one of them has it under control — 75 percent don't. This is a tragic situation!

And high blood pressure affects women of all ages:

✔ As a result of high blood pressure, *preeclampsia* and *eclampsia* are two extremely dangerous disorders that can begin in the 20th week of a pregnancy. Ignoring them raises great risks to the mother and the growing fetus.

✔ Estrogen may play an important role in women who are postmenopausal with high blood pressure. Estrogen replacement therapy can lower blood pressure in these women by as much as 10/5 mm Hg.

✔ Fifty percent of all white women and 80 percent of all black women in the United States over age 60 have high blood pressure.

✔ Women in their 70s and 80s represent a large proportion of the people with high blood pressure at that age. These women suffer heart attacks and brain attacks at a much higher rate when their high blood pressure isn't controlled.

Chapter 19

Ten New Discoveries about High Blood Pressure

*W*hen I searched *high blood pressure* at the National Library of Medicine's Web site and limited it to articles published from 1/1/2005 to 3/24/2007, I had 12,265 hits — all articles about high blood pressure that the library had catalogued from all the medical and scientific journals in the world. When I changed the search term to *hypertension,* I found 21,443 separate publications.

This great number of articles published in a little over two years indicates the enormous amount of research going on to help doctors and patients understand and treat high blood pressure. Perhaps one of these publications can solve your problem and its complications; perhaps a cure for your high blood pressure is just around the corner. But until then, you can benefit from the discoveries of thousands of people around the world making their contribution to understanding high blood pressure. This chapter provides ten new discoveries — a small sample of the published work.

You can check the literature yourself. It's simple and free on the National Center for Biotechnology Information Web site: www.ncbi.nlm.nih.gov/entrez. Type *high blood pressure* or *hypertension* in the search box and be prepared to spend a few days reading.

An inevitable (and essential) lag exists between research and publication so that scientists and researchers can verify the information before it reaches the public. To offset this lag, I provide an appendix at the end of this book that lists resources for the latest information.

Gauging the Effect of Lowering Blood Pressure

Is all the effort, time, and money that I suggest you put into lowering your blood pressure worth it? A study in the February 2005 issue of *Vascular Health Risk Management* gives a strong affirmative vote to this question. The authors studied disease-free survival of treated and untreated individuals in the United States. They found that "for a 40-year-old man, the gain in life expectancy without stroke or major cardiovascular events were 27 and 32 months" for the treated compared to the untreated individual.

Is it worth it to you to have an additional 2 years or more to spend with your children, your spouse, and your other loved ones? You bet it is!

When you control your high blood pressure, the end definitely justifies the means. Although you don't feel the difference as you exercise (see Chapter 12), follow the DASH diet (see Chapter 9), and avoid salt (see Chapter 10), your body is not being damaged as it would be without these life changes.

Realizing that Prehypertension Isn't Benign

Is prehypertension (see Chapter 2) harmless as long as it doesn't develop into high blood pressure? Unfortunately, a study by George Washington University in the February 2007 journal *Circulation* indicates that lifestyle changes are necessary even if your prehypertension never becomes high blood pressure. (See Part III for these changes.) This study followed 60,785 postmenopausal women for 7.7 years.

The percentages of women who had prehypertension at the beginning of the study were as follows: Caucasian, 39.5 percent; African American, 32.1 percent; Hispanic, 42.6 percent; American Indian, 38.7 percent; Asian, 40.3 percent.

At the end of the study:

- ✔ The women with prehypertension were about twice as likely to have a heart attack or a stroke compared with the women who did not have prehypertension.

- ✔ The women with prehypertension were about one and a half times more likely to die of heart disease than women who didn't have prehypertension.

Note: The Hispanic and Asian women had very few of these events compared to the others.

The conclusion? Prehypertension is common, and it is associated with increased heart attacks, strokes, and death due to heart attacks. (Chapter 5 has more information on heart attacks; Chapter 7 has more on strokes.)

Predicting (And Preventing) High Blood Pressure

Can you control some risk factors that predict high blood pressure? A study reported in the March 2007 *Journal of Hypertension* attempted to answer this important question by tracking 10,525 Chinese adults over an eight-year period. By the end of the study, 29 percent of the men and 27 percent of the women had developed high blood pressure. The men had several factors that predicted the onset of high blood pressure, including

- Being older
- Living in cities
- Drinking excessive amounts of alcohol
- Having less physical activity

Women were different in several respects:

- Women who smoked were more likely to have high blood pressure than those who drank.
- Women living in rural areas were more likely to have high blood pressure than city women.

The key result of this study is that nearly 50 percent of risk factors that lead to high blood pressure are modifiable (see Chapter 3 for additional info on other risk factors).

Another important lesson in prevention is in the April 2007 *American Journal of Public Health.* A study looked at the physical activity in young adults and the occurrence of high blood pressure over 15 years. Almost 4,000 young black and white men and women aged 18 to 30 years without high blood pressure were examined at the beginning of the study and then 2, 5, 7, 10, and 15 years later. Blood pressure and physical activity were recorded each time. After 15 years, 634 of them (16 percent) had high blood pressure. The people who did limited physical activity were much more likely to have high blood pressure than those who did regular physical exercise.

If you want to help your child avoid high blood pressure later in life, set an example by doing some physical activity for at least 30 minutes a day, and take your child along. See Chapter 15 for more information.

Predicting Adult High Blood Pressure by Measuring Childhood Blood Pressure

Can you predict an adult's high blood pressure by measuring her blood pressure in early childhood? One study's answer (in the February 2007 *Pediatrics*) is "Yes." The study tracked the blood pressure of 240 men and 253 women for decades, beginning at age 5. The results were the following:

- ✔ If a single measurement of systolic — but not diastolic — blood pressure exceeded the desirable levels when they were children, the probability that they would have high blood pressure as adults increased four to five times.

- ✔ The more times the blood pressure exceeded that range, the more likely they would have high blood pressure later in life.

The study clearly showed that children with blood pressures above the level suggested in this paper could expect to have high blood pressure later. But these findings don't mean you're doomed. Try to alter all the modifiable risk factors like diet, exercise, meditation, alcohol, and smoking (as I explain in Part III). You'll be glad you did.

Determining Whether All Stroke Patients Have High Blood Pressure

Without question, high blood pressure is a major cause of brain attacks. So scientists question whether high blood pressure is present in every case. In a large study published in the January 2007 *American Journal of Emergency Medicine,* the authors looked at 563,704 emergency patients with acute brain attacks.

A total of 69 percent of those patients had high blood pressure initially:

- ✔ 56 percent were between 140 and 184 mm Hg.

- ✔ 13 percent were between 185 and 219 mm Hg.

- ✔ Only 0.1 percent were 220 mm Hg or above.

Is there any doubt in your mind that high blood pressure causes brain attacks? If you still have questions, flip to Chapter 7 for more information.

Evaluating the Effect of Job Strain

It's not clear whether *job strain* (where a person has a very demanding job but very little decision-making latitude) increases the tendency to have high blood pressure. The March 2007 *Journal of Hypertension* reported a study of 448 men and women with a mean age of 55 who were followed for 6.5 years. Their blood pressure was checked and the demands of their work were measured. The study concluded:

- ✔ For men: The demands of work seemed to have more effect on blood pressure than the amount of decision-making latitude.

- ✔ For women: Neither the demands of work nor the amount of decision-making latitude were associated with high blood pressure.

If you're a man who suffers from a lot of job strain and you have high blood pressure, a less demanding job will have a positive effect upon your blood pressure. If you're a woman in the same situation, changing your job probably won't make a difference in your blood pressure — although it'll certainly make life more enjoyable. Head to Chapter 8 for an introduction to steps you can take to lower your stress (such as including more humor in your life).

Knowing Whether Alcohol Is Good or Bad if You Have High Blood Pressure

It's well known that *heavy* alcohol consumption increases the risk for high blood pressure, which increases the risk for heart disease (see Chapter 11 for details). However, can a person with high blood pressure safely consume a *small amount* of alcohol?

A group at the Harvard School of Public Health published their findings on this subject in the January 2007 *Annals of Internal Medicine*. They had studied 11,711 men with high blood pressure for six years, comparing the men who didn't drink at all with the men who consumed small amounts of alcohol. During those years, 653 heart attacks occurred. The results showed:

- ✔ The men who drank moderately (one to two glasses of wine a night, maximum of ten a week) had a significantly lower risk of a heart attack.

- ✔ The men who drank moderately did not have a lower death rate overall.

The overall death rate for those who drank moderately was not lower probably because of other causes such as brain attacks.

Using Gastric Bypass to Lower Weight and Blood Pressure

Is there a role for gastric bypass in the treatment of high blood pressure? A paper in the February 2007 *Nutrition in Clinical Practice* presented the results for 400 consecutive gastric-bypass patients after a year post-op, looking specifically at diabetes, arthritis, high blood pressure, gastroesophageal reflux (where stomach acids reenter the esophagus causing severe pain), asthma, and depression.

The results showed:

- ✔ At six weeks, over 35 percent of the patients had greatly improved their quality of life; by the end of the year, over 80 percent had greatly improved their quality of life.

- ✔ Most of the abnormalities, including blood pressure, improved 80 to 100 percent by the end of the year.

- ✔ Arthritis and depression did not improve as much, only 50 to 75 percent.

These excellent responses to weight loss may not be permanent. A number of patients regain a lot of their weight, and the complications naturally follow. However, even if you control your blood pressure for only one year, that's one less year of damage to your body. And because the complications only increase with higher blood pressure, any control is desirable.

Checking Whether Your Blood Pressure Drug Affects Diabetes

Doctors and scientist recognize that several blood pressure medications tend to bring out diabetes. (The meds don't seem to cause diabetes, but they raise the blood sugar to a diabetic level in a patient who is *prediabetic,* that is, predisposed to adult-onset diabetes.) However, it has been difficult to determine how each class of drugs compares with the others in its tendency to raise the blood sugar level.

To address the problem, a study published in the January 2007 *Lancet* looked at 143,153 patients to determine the proportion of patients who developed diabetes only after they started on a specific drug.

The following list rates drugs from least likely to bring out diabetes to most likely:

- ✔ ACE inhibitors and angiotensin receptor blockers
- ✔ Calcium channel blockers
- ✔ *Placebos* (drugs containing no active ingredients in order to assess the performance of a new drug)
- ✔ Beta blockers
- ✔ Diuretics

Because ACE inhibitors, angiotensin receptor blockers, and calcium channel blockers were even less likely than placebos to bring out diabetes, the authors determined that these drugs are not associated with diabetes at all.

Does this mean you shouldn't use diuretics? As I point out many times in Chapter 13, diuretics remain the first choice for blood pressure control.

Considering the Significance of the ALLHAT Study

The Antihypertensive and Lipid Lowering Treatment to Prevent Heart Attack Trial (ALLHAT Study), published in the December 2002 *Journal of the American Medical Association,* was the largest clinical study up to that time. It followed 40,000 patients over five years. The patients took different blood pressure medications in increasing doses until they achieved the target blood pressure of less than 140/90. A second drug was added when necessary. The major findings of that study were as follows:

- ✔ 60 percent of patients reached the goal of less than 140/90.
- ✔ Compared to the other drugs, the diuretic *chlorthalidone* (see Chapter 13) at a low dose (which is not generally associated with side effects like raised blood sugar and impotency) proved to be best at lowering blood pressure and preventing heart attacks.

The findings of the ALLHAT Study were so conclusive that it should have caused a definite change in drug usage. But did it? A paper in the December 2006 *Journal of Clinical Hypertension* showed that the study did make a difference in the prescribing habits of doctors. Researchers studied two groups with high blood pressure, one was from a year before the paper and the other was a year after the paper. The results showed

✔ Before the study, 29 percent of new high blood pressure patients were started on thiazide diuretics, of which chlorthalidone is an example.

✔ Just a year after the study, 39 percent of new patients were started on thiazide diuretics.

This increase in diuretic treatment is really an amazing response, considering the usual speed with which physicians change when studies clearly show a different treatment is appropriate.

Another question from the ALLHAT Study was whether chlorthalidone was really superior to the other drugs in the prevention of heart failure because several reviewers of the study claimed that the diagnosis of heart failure was not made correctly. As a result, a follow-up study was performed to validate the first study, with its results published in the January 2007 *American Heart Journal*. The second study conclusively showed almost complete agreement between the physicians who originally made a diagnosis of heart failure and reviewers who looked at the diagnosis some time later.

The conclusion of the second study was the same as that in the original ALLHAT paper: All the other classes of drugs used as the first step in treatment of high blood pressure have a higher occurrence of heart failure when compared to the diuretic chlorthalidone.

Unless a doctor has a very good reason for using another drug as the first step in treating high blood pressure (such as kidney disease in diabetes; see Chapter 13), a low-dose diuretic is the treatment of first choice in every case.

Appendix

Resources for the Latest Information

A wealth of information about high blood pressure is waiting for you. If you think the riches that the old pirates left on some Caribbean island are vast, just wait until you tap into the riches that many organizations and people provide free of charge about high blood pressure. It boggles the mind. And practically all of it's on the Internet. You can read it, download it, print it out, or just stare at it happily. What? You still don't have a connection to the Internet? If you have high blood pressure, the Internet treasures on this subject alone are enough reason to get connected.

However, if you've decided to live and die without ever touching a computer keyboard, another means is still available for accessing valuable information on high blood pressure — that quaint instrument, the telephone. And if all else fails, you have the phenomenon called *snail mail* — anything that's carried from place to place. When available, I provide you with an organization's phone number and address in addition to the Web site.

How do you know whether a Web site offers authoritative information or unsubstantiated myths? Fortunately, Health On the Net Foundation (HON), an international Swiss organization, has made it their mission to help people like you and me access valid medical and health-related information on the Web. Any site with the HON logo has fulfilled the requirements of the HON Code of Conduct:

- ✔ Only qualified individuals offer medical advice.
- ✔ The user's identity is kept confidential.
- ✔ Claims of medical treatment are supported by evidence.
- ✔ Advertising and editorial information are clearly separated.

HON recognizes all the Web sites in this chapter. However, if you want to search for its links to other medical topics, go to their index page (www.hon.ch) and enter your keyword. After you click Search, the next page lets you limit your search to those sites subscribing to the HON Code. For example, using the keyword *hypertension,* the site showed a total of 3,081 resources on high blood pressure: 152 sites subscribed to the code; 13,282 sites didn't. My advice? Stick with the first group.

National Heart, Lung, and Blood Institute

The National Heart, Lung, and Blood Institutes's Web site (www.nhlbi.nih.gov/hbp) is a great resource for understanding more about high blood pressure. (You can also reach the program at 301-592-8573 or write to NHLBI Health Information Center, Attention: Web Site, P.O. Box 30105, Bethesda, MD 20824-0105.) In 1972, the institute began creating public education programs to assist in the reduction of high blood pressure and its complications.

This site has also many resources concerning high blood pressure. On the index page, you can find 55 topics — from ACE inhibitors to hormone replacement therapy to the white coat effect and everything in between. Besides the basic information, this site includes tips and quizzes, information about medications and working with your doctor, and real-life examples of people with high blood pressure.

If you want additional information, click Contact NHLBI and follow the links for an answer to just about any question on high blood pressure.

For information on the National High Blood Pressure Education Month (each May), check out http://hin.nhlbi.nih.gov/nhbpep_kit.

American Society of Hypertension

In 1985, a group of professionals who wanted to organize and promote the advancement of scientific information related to cardiovascular diseases started the American Society of Hypertension, now an organization of over 3,000 medical professionals.

The organization's Web site (www.ash-us.org) offers extensive information about high blood pressure. Although the society doesn't make any recommendations, their site provides the names and addresses of specialists in the clinical treatment of high blood pressure who are members of the organization.

You can also write to the American Society of Hypertension at 148 Madison Avenue, 5th Floor, New York, NY 10016, or call 212-696-9099.

The society's pamphlet *Understanding Hypertension* is available from the Internet or by writing to the organization. Other important publications from the American Society of Hypertension include the *American Journal of Hypertension* and *Current Concepts in Clinical Hypertension,* a newsletter; both are directed toward the professional.

National Kidney Foundation

The kidneys are among those major organs that may contribute to high blood pressure *and* be damaged by it (see Chapter 6 for more information). The National Kidney Foundation's Web site (www.kidney.org) has important information on the kidneys in general and specific help regarding high blood pressure and kidneys. You can also write to the National Kidney Foundation at 30 East 33rd Street, New York, NY 10016 or call 800-622-9010.

The site contains information on several categories such as health information, donor family support, nutrition, treatment, rehabilitation, organ donation, and healthcare services. If you choose *kidney disease,* for example, the site provides about 40 topics that cover every aspect of disease affecting the kidneys. Many of the topics deal with both high blood pressure and kidney disease.

The National Kidney Foundation also publishes three magazines: *Family Focus* for dialysis patients; *Transplant Chronicles* for people who have received a kidney transplant; and *For Those Who Give and Grieve,* a publication for loved ones of organ donors. (Subscribe to these publications by writing to the National Kidney Foundation at the address earlier in this section.)

National Institute of Diabetes and Digestive and Kidney Diseases

The National Institute of Diabetes and Digestive and Kidney Diseases Web site (www.niddk.nih.gov) has valuable information on all aspects of diabetes, gastrointestinal disease, and kidney disease. You can access information specific to high blood pressure and the kidneys at http://kidney.niddk.nih.gov. This area of the site provides answers for how high blood pressure damages the kidneys, how you can prevent it, and what to do if kidney damage has already occurred. (See Chapter 6 for more information about the effect of high blood pressure on kidneys.)

The site also links to numerous publications on all aspects of kidney diseases (for example, you can find extensive descriptions of dialysis techniques).

To request information through the mail, write to National Kidney and Urologic Diseases Information Clearinghouse, 3 Information Way, Bethesda, MD 20892–3580. You can call them at 800–891–5390.

The organization also offers many of its publications in Spanish.

American Heart and Stroke Associations

The American Stroke Association (www.strokeassociation.org) is a division of the American Heart Association (www.americanheart.org). Both associations' Web sites offer extensive information for professionals and patients, providing thousands of pages of information and links to other resources for high blood pressure and brain attacks (see Chapter 7 for details on brain attacks).

You can write to the American Heart Association or the American Stroke Association for more information at 7272 Greenville Avenue, Dallas, TX 75231 — they use the same address. The American Heart Association's phone number is 800-242-8721 and the American Stroke Association's phone number is 888-478-7653.

American Heart Association

The New York Heart Association was formed in 1915 by a group of physicians in New York City who were dedicated to gathering and expanding the available information on heart disease. In 1924, similar groups throughout the country joined with New York group to form the American Heart Association. Although it had started as a scientific society, in 1948 the association transformed itself into an agency of professional and nonprofessional volunteers. Its mission is to reduce complications from cardiovascular disease and stroke.

Although some advertisements get in the way in this site, they are clearly differentiated from the excellent medical information (for example, a series of questions and their extensive answers about high blood pressure). In addition, the site carries stories of people who have survived brain attacks, and it publishes statistics on every aspect of heart disease.

American Stroke Association

The American Stroke Association Web site offers information about the prevention of brain attacks (see Chapter 7), caring for the person who has a brain attack, medical resources, and just about anything you need to know for dealing with this high blood pressure complication.

This site also features pen pals so a brain attack sufferer can communicate with another person who has had a similar attack. To get to that feature from the main page, click Life After Stroke in the left column, then Getting Support, then Stroke Family Warmline. Finally, under Related Items on the right side of this page, click Common Threads Pen Pals.

Along with the Web site, the American Stroke Association publishes *Stroke Connection Magazine* that contains articles for people recovering from a brain attack. If you don't have Web access, you can write to the American Stroke Association (I give the address earlier in this section) to subscribe to this magazine.

National Stroke Association

The National Stroke Association Web site (www.stroke.org) describes itself as the one nonprofit organization that's 100 percent devoted to stroke. They provide links to the most common symptoms, recovery and rehabilitation, stroke risk, the description of a stroke, acute treatment, effects of stroke, and stroke survivors and their family. I'd say that just about covers everything you need to know about brain attacks (see Chapter 7).

You can write to them at National Stroke Association, 9707 East Easter Lane, Centennial, CO 80112. Their phone number is 800-787-6537.

You can become a nonprofessional member of the organization and receive *Stroke Smart* magazine. Or, if you're a professional, you can join the Professional Society and receive the *Journal of Stroke and Cerebrovascular Disease* as well as the journal *Stroke: Clinical Updates.*

One of the most useful features of the National Stroke Association site is the link Related Web Sites and Products, where you can find just about any product for a brain attack victim: lifts, walkers, wheelchairs, elevators, ramps, reading and writing aids, products for incontinence and hygiene, special clothing, and computers and other communication devices for brain attack victims. From the association's home page, click on the following links:

- ✔ EMS/Prehospital Providers, then Find a Stroke Center and Other Resources Near You

  This link provides valuable information for the loved ones of the brain attack victim — from support groups to life at home; from dealing with rehabilitation to how the loved one can help.

- ✔ Medical Professionals, then Stroke Trials Directory (in the right column)

  This link tells you about ongoing drug studies and how you can play a role in the study if you've had a brain attack.

All in all, this site is the first place to go when you need information on any aspect of prevention, treatment, and rehabilitation for a brain attack.

United States National Library of Medicine

The United States National Library of Medicine Web site (www.nlm.nih.gov) provides links to MedlinePlus Health Information and PubMed (see the following sections). You can also write to the library for more information at 8600 Rockville Pike, Bethesda, MD 20894 or call 888-346-3656.

MedlinePlus

The MedlinePlus Web site (www.medlineplus.gov) contains about 700 discussions of health topics from the National Institutes of Health. Go to www.nlm.nih.gov/medlineplus/highbloodpressure.html for discussions specific to high blood pressure.

The MedlinePlus site contains basic descriptions of high blood pressure as well as up-to-date information about the latest discoveries and medical advances in general. When I visited, I found references to articles that had appeared in medical journals just three days earlier. MedlinePlus also provides

✔ A medical encyclopedia and dictionaries

✔ Extensive information on prescription and nonprescription drugs

✔ Health information from newspaper and magazine sources

✔ Health information in Spanish

✔ Links to thousands of clinical trials

✔ Lists of hospitals and physicians by state

Don't take my word for it, though. *Consumer Reports,* which is my Bible for reliable consumer information, voted MedlinePlus the best consumer-health Web site for dependable medical information in its January 2002 issue.

Like all government sites, MedlinePlus doesn't carry any advertisements or endorsements.

If you have an e-mail address, you can sign up for MedlinePlus weekly updates.

PubMed

You can search PubMed (www.pubmed.gov) for any medical term. In this case, type in "high blood pressure" and click Go to see thousands of references, many with short descriptions, to its related medical literature. If you want to limit your search to certain types of literature (such as reviews of a particular subject within a certain time span), click Limits and choose the appropriate limits for your search.

The PubMed site is only available online. And the fact that you can access thousands of articles on any medical topic with the touch of your finger is amazing. If you need justification for paying your federal taxes, the PubMed site serves that function well. Did I just write "justification for paying your federal taxes?" Oh, well.

The Mayo Clinic

The world-renowned Mayo Clinic has a Web site (www.mayoclinic.com) with extensive material on every aspect of disease including high blood pressure. Going to this Web site is like having a super-easy-to-understand medical textbook. By clicking Diseases & Conditions on the home page, you can find links to various other pages, other valuable Web sites, and discussions on high blood pressure.

Lifeclinic Health Management Systems

Lifeclinic Health Management Systems has extensive information about three major health disorders: high blood pressure, high cholesterol, and diabetes. Simply type the Lifeclinic Web site (www.lifeclinic.com) and explore.

Although you see some advertising, this site follows the HON Code of Conduct (I discuss this code earlier in this chapter). It goes through basic facts about high blood pressure and then how to lower it. The site explains monitoring your blood pressure and the risk factors for heart disease (see Chapter 5). You can also locate discussions on low blood pressure, high blood pressure, and pregnancy (see Chapter 16), brain attacks (see Chapter 7), and heart failure (see Chapter 5) at this site.

One of the best features of the site is a personal health record that you develop, maintain, and access (with the proper identification and password) from any computer. You can keep a health checklist as well as records of your blood pressure, pulse, weight, cholesterol, blood sugar, personal health, and family health.

If you have health questions, the site has a place for you to ask the experts. An extensive directory of medicines is also available to provide everything you need to know about a medication including its effect, adverse reactions, drug interactions, dosage information, and storage tips.

A physician directory is available as well as Web site reviews, book reviews, patient pamphlets, topics regarding high blood pressure, and the latest news. You can also find a cookbook with healthy recipes; each recipe lists its kilo-calorie sources and nutrient amounts.

Lifeclinic has 11,700 Health Stations in retail stores where you can get health information. The Web site has won numerous awards for the quality of its material. You'll benefit from its information and the many services it offers.

Other Sites

Other useful Web sites include the following:

- ✔ American Occupational Therapy Association at www.aota.org
- ✔ American Physical Therapy Association at www.apta.org
- ✔ American Speech-Language-Hearing Association at asha.org

- ✔ DASH diet at the National Institutes of Health at `www.nhlbi.nih.gov/health/public/heart/hbp/dash` (I discuss the DASH diet in detail in Chapter 9.)

- ✔ National Aphasia Association at `aphasia.org`

- ✔ National Rehabilitation Information Association at `naric.com`

- ✔ High Blood Pressure and Hypertension at `www.blood-pressure-hypertension.com`

- ✔ WebMD at `www.medscape.com/publichealth` (type "WebMD" in the search box)

If you live outside the United States, some of the best sources of information about high blood pressure are at the following addresses:

- ✔ United Kingdom: Patient UK at `www.patient.co.uk/illness/b/blood_pressure.htm`

- ✔ Australia: The National Heart Foundation of Australia at `www.heartfoundation.com.au`

- ✔ Canada: The Canadian Coalition for High Blood Pressure Prevention and Control at `www.canadianbpcoalition.org/english/links.htm`

- ✔ Other countries: The World Hypertension League at `www.worldhypertensionleague.org`

Index

• *I* •

BUSINESS, CAREERS & PERSONAL FINANCE

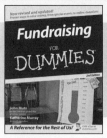

0-7645-9847-3

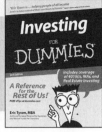

0-7645-2431-3

Also available:
- Business Plans Kit For Dummies
  0-7645-9794-9
- Economics For Dummies
  0-7645-5726-2
- Grant Writing For Dummies
  0-7645-8416-2
- Home Buying For Dummies
  0-7645-5331-3
- Managing For Dummies
  0-7645-1771-6
- Marketing For Dummies
  0-7645-5600-2

- Personal Finance For Dummies
  0-7645-2590-5*
- Resumes For Dummies
  0-7645-5471-9
- Selling For Dummies
  0-7645-5363-1
- Six Sigma For Dummies
  0-7645-6798-5
- Small Business Kit For Dummies
  0-7645-5984-2
- Starting an eBay Business For Dummies
  0-7645-6924-4
- Your Dream Career For Dummies
  0-7645-9795-7

HOME & BUSINESS COMPUTER BASICS

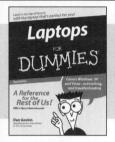

0-470-05432-8

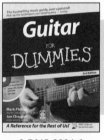

0-471-75421-8

Also available:
- Cleaning Windows Vista For Dummies
  0-471-78293-9
- Excel 2007 For Dummies
  0-470-03737-7
- Mac OS X Tiger For Dummies
  0-7645-7675-5
- MacBook For Dummies
  0-470-04859-X
- Macs For Dummies
  0-470-04849-2
- Office 2007 For Dummies
  0-470-00923-3

- Outlook 2007 For Dummies
  0-470-03830-6
- PCs For Dummies
  0-7645-8958-X
- Salesforce.com For Dummies
  0-470-04893-X
- Upgrading & Fixing Laptops For Dummies
  0-7645-8959-8
- Word 2007 For Dummies
  0-470-03658-3
- Quicken 2007 For Dummies
  0-470-04600-7

FOOD, HOME, GARDEN, HOBBIES, MUSIC & PETS

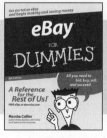

0-7645-8404-9

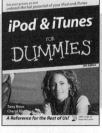

0-7645-9904-6

Also available:
- Candy Making For Dummies
  0-7645-9734-5
- Card Games For Dummies
  0-7645-9910-0
- Crocheting For Dummies
  0-7645-4151-X
- Dog Training For Dummies
  0-7645-8418-9
- Healthy Carb Cookbook For Dummies
  0-7645-8476-6
- Home Maintenance For Dummies
  0-7645-5215-5

- Horses For Dummies
  0-7645-9797-3
- Jewelry Making & Beading For Dummies
  0-7645-2571-9
- Orchids For Dummies
  0-7645-6759-4
- Puppies For Dummies
  0-7645-5255-4
- Rock Guitar For Dummies
  0-7645-5356-9
- Sewing For Dummies
  0-7645-6847-7
- Singing For Dummies
  0-7645-2475-5

INTERNET & DIGITAL MEDIA

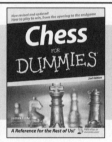

0-470-04529-9

0-470-04894-8

Also available:
- Blogging For Dummies
  0-471-77084-1
- Digital Photography For Dummies
  0-7645-9802-3
- Digital Photography All-in-One Desk Reference For Dummies
  0-470-03743-1
- Digital SLR Cameras and Photography For Dummies
  0-7645-9803-1
- eBay Business All-in-One Desk Reference For Dummies
  0-7645-8438-3
- HDTV For Dummies
  0-470-09673-X

- Home Entertainment PCs For Dummies
  0-470-05523-5
- MySpace For Dummies
  0-470-09529-6
- Search Engine Optimization For Dummies
  0-471-97998-8
- Skype For Dummies
  0-470-04891-3
- The Internet For Dummies
  0-7645-8996-2
- Wiring Your Digital Home For Dummies
  0-471-91830-X

* Separate Canadian edition also available
† Separate U.K. edition also available

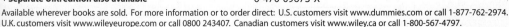

Available wherever books are sold. For more information or to order direct: U.S. customers visit www.dummies.com or call 1-877-762-2974.
U.K. customers visit www.wileyeurope.com or call 0800 243407. Canadian customers visit www.wiley.ca or call 1-800-567-4797.

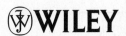 **WILEY**

SPORTS, FITNESS, PARENTING, RELIGION & SPIRITUALITY

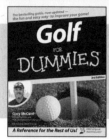

0-471-76871-5

0-7645-7841-3

Also available:

- Catholicism For Dummies
  0-7645-5391-7
- Exercise Balls For Dummies
  0-7645-5623-1
- Fitness For Dummies
  0-7645-7851-0
- Football For Dummies
  0-7645-3936-1
- Judaism For Dummies
  0-7645-5299-6
- Potty Training For Dummies
  0-7645-5417-4
- Buddhism For Dummies
  0-7645-5359-3

- Pregnancy For Dummies
  0-7645-4483-7 †
- Ten Minute Tone-Ups For Dummies
  0-7645-7207-5
- NASCAR For Dummies
  0-7645-7681-X
- Religion For Dummies
  0-7645-5264-3
- Soccer For Dummies
  0-7645-5229-5
- Women in the Bible For Dummies
  0-7645-8475-8

TRAVEL

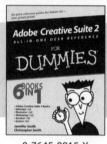

0-7645-7749-2

0-7645-6945-7

Also available:

- Alaska For Dummies
  0-7645-7746-8
- Cruise Vacations For Dummies
  0-7645-6941-4
- England For Dummies
  0-7645-4276-1
- Europe For Dummies
  0-7645-7529-5
- Germany For Dummies
  0-7645-7823-5
- Hawaii For Dummies
  0-7645-7402-7

- Italy For Dummies
  0-7645-7386-1
- Las Vegas For Dummies
  0-7645-7382-9
- London For Dummies
  0-7645-4277-X
- Paris For Dummies
  0-7645-7630-5
- RV Vacations For Dummies
  0-7645-4442-X
- Walt Disney World & Orlando
  For Dummies
  0-7645-9660-8

GRAPHICS, DESIGN & WEB DEVELOPMENT

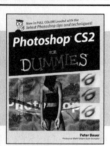

0-7645-8815-X

0-7645-9571-7

Also available:

- 3D Game Animation For Dummies
  0-7645-8789-7
- AutoCAD 2006 For Dummies
  0-7645-8925-3
- Building a Web Site For Dummies
  0-7645-7144-3
- Creating Web Pages For Dummies
  0-470-08030-2
- Creating Web Pages All-in-One Desk
  Reference For Dummies
  0-7645-4345-8
- Dreamweaver 8 For Dummies
  0-7645-9649-7

- InDesign CS2 For Dummies
  0-7645-9572-5
- Macromedia Flash 8 For Dummies
  0-7645-9691-8
- Photoshop CS2 and Digital
  Photography For Dummies
  0-7645-9580-6
- Photoshop Elements 4 For Dummies
  0-471-77483-9
- Syndicating Web Sites with RSS Feeds
  For Dummies
  0-7645-8848-6
- Yahoo! SiteBuilder For Dummies
  0-7645-9800-7

NETWORKING, SECURITY, PROGRAMMING & DATABASES

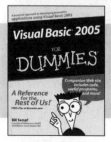

0-7645-7728-X

0-471-74940-0

Also available:

- Access 2007 For Dummies
  0-470-04612-0
- ASP.NET 2 For Dummies
  0-7645-7907-X
- C# 2005 For Dummies
  0-7645-9704-3
- Hacking For Dummies
  0-470-05235-X
- Hacking Wireless Networks
  For Dummies
  0-7645-9730-2
- Java For Dummies
  0-470-08716-1

- Microsoft SQL Server 2005 For Dummies
  0-7645-7755-7
- Networking All-in-One Desk Reference
  For Dummies
  0-7645-9939-9
- Preventing Identity Theft For Dummies
  0-7645-7336-5
- Telecom For Dummies
  0-471-77085-X
- Visual Studio 2005 All-in-One Desk
  Reference For Dummies
  0-7645-9775-2
- XML For Dummies
  0-7645-8845-1

HEALTH & SELF-HELP

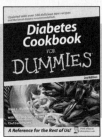

0-7645-8450-2

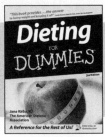

0-7645-4149-8

Also available:
- Bipolar Disorder For Dummies
  0-7645-8451-0
- Chemotherapy and Radiation
  For Dummies
  0-7645-7832-4
- Controlling Cholesterol For Dummies
  0-7645-5440-9
- Diabetes For Dummies
  0-7645-6820-5* †
- Divorce For Dummies
  0-7645-8417-0 †

- Fibromyalgia For Dummies
  0-7645-5441-7
- Low-Calorie Dieting For Dummies
  0-7645-9905-4
- Meditation For Dummies
  0-471-77774-9
- Osteoporosis For Dummies
  0-7645-7621-6
- Overcoming Anxiety For Dummies
  0-7645-5447-6
- Reiki For Dummies
  0-7645-9907-0
- Stress Management For Dummies
  0-7645-5144-2

EDUCATION, HISTORY, REFERENCE & TEST PREPARATION

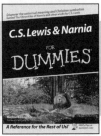

0-7645-8381-6

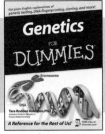

0-7645-9554-7

Also available:
- The ACT For Dummies
  0-7645-9652-7
- Algebra For Dummies
  0-7645-5325-9
- Algebra Workbook For Dummies
  0-7645-8467-7
- Astronomy For Dummies
  0-7645-8465-0
- Calculus For Dummies
  0-7645-2498-4
- Chemistry For Dummies
  0-7645-5430-1
- Forensics For Dummies
  0-7645-5580-4

- Freemasons For Dummies
  0-7645-9796-5
- French For Dummies
  0-7645-5193-0
- Geometry For Dummies
  0-7645-5324-0
- Organic Chemistry I For Dummies
  0-7645-6902-3
- The SAT I For Dummies
  0-7645-7193-1
- Spanish For Dummies
  0-7645-5194-9
- Statistics For Dummies
  0-7645-5423-9

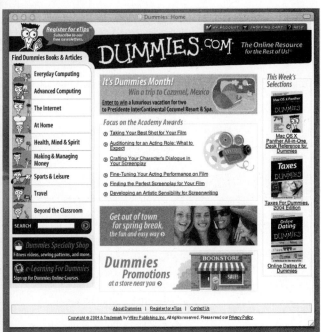

Get smart @ dummies.com®

- **Find a full list of Dummies titles**
- **Look into loads of FREE on-site articles**
- **Sign up for FREE eTips e-mailed to you weekly**
- **See what other products carry the Dummies name**
- **Shop directly from the Dummies bookstore**
- **Enter to win new prizes every month!**

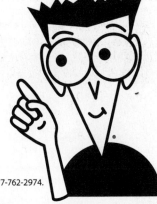

* Separate Canadian edition also available

† Separate U.K. edition also available

Available wherever books are sold. For more information or to order direct: U.S. customers visit www.dummies.com or call 1-877-762-2974.
U.K. customers visit www.wileyeurope.com or call 0800 243407. Canadian customers visit www.wiley.ca or call 1-800-567-4797.

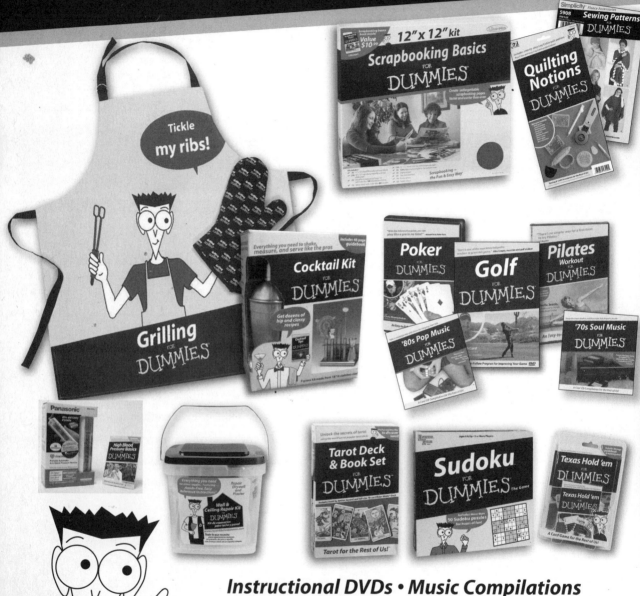

Do More with Dummies

Instructional DVDs • Music Compilations
Games & Novelties • Culinary Kits
Crafts & Sewing Patterns
Home Improvement/DIY Kits • and more!

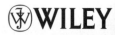